The BMS Ecosystem

GROW INTO YOUR EXCELLENCE

By

Dr. Harris E. Phillip

Dedication

To my children Brandon, Kyle, Hillery, and Chantel whose lives I have tried to steer with the principles contained in this book.

In memory of my loving and caring parents, Burnham and Blanche Phillip, who doubtlessly sowed the seeds, which germinated and blossomed into who I am today.

Foreword

Dear reader…

Do you feel that you try to take care of yourself the best way you know how but always feel that you fall short of your desired energy levels?

Have you ever wondered what the secret to a life full of energy is?

Perhaps you feel that something is missing, or you are constantly struggling to find a sense of balance.

We all want to live a long and healthy life. But what good is a long life if it is not filled with the energy you need to make it your best life? Dr. Harris Phillip has not only been practicing medicine for more than 30 years but has also been fascinated by how to create not only a long life but also a vibrant life. This is his life's passion, and he is ready to share it with the world.

He has developed a clear pathway to finding balance and wants this information to now be yours. Not only does his precise observations and reflections make it doable, it is accessible to every one of us no matter where we are in life. Dr. Phillip takes the ideas of our body, mind, and spirit, and breaks them down into clear and manageable components of our Self. He will guide you on how to nurture not only each component from the inside out but also the outside in.

If you find this book in your hand, it may be a sign from the Universe that you are ready to live the life you have always dreamed of. It is never too late to make changes and delve deeper into the relationship of your body, mind, and spirit. Let Dr. Phillip remind you that all the tools you need are within arm's reach, and you can reap the benefits of reviving your body, mind, and spirit.

Loral Langemeier

The Millionaire Maker

Introduction

"Not life, but good life is to be chiefly valued." – *Socrates*

Have you reached a point on your journey where you feel your life is at a standstill? You feel you've reached some sort of peak and that there is nowhere left to go but down... It is not too late to start living a fuller, more productive, and vibrant life! It is not too late to add years to your life and, in the process, grow into your excellence. How can you achieve this, and why is it such a secret?

Humans are a triune. We are more complex than just our physical bodies. We are made of three distinct components: Body, Mind, and Spirit. Each component has its own unique characteristics, and all three together create a functioning unit: a human being. Each component (the body, mind, and spirit) must be looked after individually to ensure productive and enjoyable years are added to your lives. You can view how to care for each component from the perspective of how you nourish it, what environment you surround it with, and what you allow to impact it. That is what the **BMS Ecosystem** is all about. I want to take you through each component and empower you with the appreciation of the value of nourishing yourself appropriately, the environment in which you are nourishing yourself, and finally, bring awareness to what you are allowing to impact you and stand in your way of growing into your excellence.

You will be awarded the tools necessary to integrate all three components of yourself and come to fully understand that through appropriate care, you will add years to your life and life to your years while growing into your excellence! In the words of Albert Einstein: "Nothing happens until something moves." It is not too late to make something happen, so please make these necessary changes for yourself, so you can start moving by reaping the rewards and grow into your excellence. Let us dive in!

Table of Contents

Dedication iii

Foreword iv

Introduction vi

Section 1: The Body 1

Chapter 1: Nourishing the Body 2

    The Food 2

    Macronutrient #1: Carbohydrates 3

    Macronutrient #2: Fats 5

    Sources of Saturated Fats 6

    Macronutrient #3: Proteins 8

    Reflection: 11

Chapter 2: Source of Food 12

    Types of Food 12

    Carnivore Diet 13

    Beef and other Red Processed Meats 15

    Types of Plant-Based Diets 16

    Virtues of a Vegetarian Diet 17

    Inflammation 17

    Microbiome 18

The Best Self-caring Diet 19

My Personal Experience 21

Hydration 22

Reflection: 24

Chapter 3: Nutrition versus Nourishment 26

The Difference 26

Proteins, Fats, and Carbohydrates: Nutrition, not necessarily
Nourishment 26

Micronutrients 29

Water 29

Chlorine in Our Water Supply 31

Reflection: 33

Chapter 4: Our Environment 35

The Environmental Challenges 35

Air 35

Sunlight 40

Reflection: 42

Chapter 5: Factors That Impact Your Body 43

Controllable Factors 43

Benefits of Physical Exercise 43

Types of Exercise and the Importance of Intensity 45

Reflection: 48

The Importance of Rest 49

Sleep 51

Reflection: 54

Temperance 55

Reflection 57

PART TWO: THE MIND 59

Chapter 6: An Introduction to Your Mind 62

The Mind 62

The Parable of Talents 65

Reflection: 68

The Influences of The Mind 69

Overcoming the Ego 71

Reflection: 73

Chapter 7: Boxed In 74

Entrapment 74

The Phenomenon of Tiptoeing 76

The Power of Praise 78

Reflections: 80

Chapter 8: The Tentacles of our Creation 81

    The Dynamic 81

    In Sports 82

    Character versus Mindset 85

    Staying on Top 85

    Success versus Failure – A Mindset Perspective 86

    Mindset and Team Dynamics 87

    Mindset in Business and Leadership 87

    ORGANIZATIONAL MINDSET 89

    Does Mindset Affect Relationships? 90

    Reflection: 95

Chapter 9: The Birth and Cultivation of Mindsets 97

    The Beginnings 97

    Addressing Failure 101

    Is Discipline Teaching? 103

    Is there a False Growth Mindset? 104

    Reflection 107

Chapter 10: Nourishment of the Mind 108

    Not Discernable by Our Senses 108

    Fixed Mindset and Growth Mindset 109

The Repair of a Fixed Mindset and Nourishing a Growth Mindset
....112

The Dangers of a Fixed Mindset.................................114

Reflection:...116

Chapter 11: The Effect of the Environment on Your Mind.................118

The Mind and its Environment.................................118

Neutralizing a Hostile Environment.................................119

Nourishing "Food" for the Mind.................................120

My Story...122

Reflection:...126

Chapter 12: Impacting the Mind.................................128

The Mind...128

Bad Habits...129

Limiting Beliefs...129

Reflection:...131

Fear...132

Reflection:...134

Boredom...134

Reflection:...137

Stress...137

Reflection:..139

Chapter 13: Changing Mindsets 141

The Challenge 141

The Change 143

Developing the Growth Mindset 145

Entitlement: The Problem 146

The Process 147

PART 3: THE SPIRIT 149

Chapter 14: The Human Spirit 150

The Spirit 150

Emotion 153

The Role of Your Spirit 155

Faith 156

Visualization and Faith 160

Reflection:..165

Chapter 15: Nourishing Your Spirit 167

Feeding the Spirit...167

The Emotional Guidance System (EGS) 168

Doubt and Disappointment....................................173

Reflection:..175

Happiness...176

Relationship Breakdown...177

Wellbeing 179

Reflection:..181

Chapter 16: Nurturing Your spirit 182

Steps..182

Negative people 182

Internal Negativity 185

Natural Laws and the Law of Attraction.........................189

The Flow...191

Reflection:..193

Chapter 17: Impact on Our Spirit......................................195

Understanding the Spirit..195

Revisiting the Emotional Guidance System (EGS) 195

The EGS at Work...197

Reflection:..200

Chapter 18: Belief and Faith 201

The Impact of Belief...201

Faith and the EGS...201

Reflection:..202

Coping Mechanisms 204

Reflection: 207

Chapter 19: Stress Management 208

Defining Stress 208

Types of Stress 208

The Stress Cycle 209

Is Stress Management Important? 210

Chronic Stress 211

Exhaustion and its Sequelae 212

The 6R Syndicate 212

Reflection: 214

Chapter 20: Journaling – The Focus Intensifier 215

Journaling 215

Gratitude Journaling 217

Thoughts and Their Triggers 218

Negative Self-Talk 218

Planful Time Management 220

Reflection: 221

Chapter 21: Bringing It All Together 222

The Complexity 222

Reflection: 225

Final Thoughts 226

Acknowledgements 229

Biography – Long 231

Biography – Short 232

Section 1: The Body

"The body politic, as well as the human body, begins to die as soon as it is born, and carries itself the causes of destruction." – Jean-Jacques Rousseau

Your physical body is one part of the overly complex structure that makes up the human being. The approach to revival of us tends to focus heavily on just the body and not so much on the other equally important components of the triune, the mind and spirit. We will cover those later in the book. I want to focus initially on the physical body. As the American psychologist Abraham Maslow contends, we need to first address our physiological needs before our other needs are met. Maslow was able to structure human needs into a pyramid. He believed that our basic physiological needs form the base of the pyramid, and these needs must first be met before other needs are fulfilled.

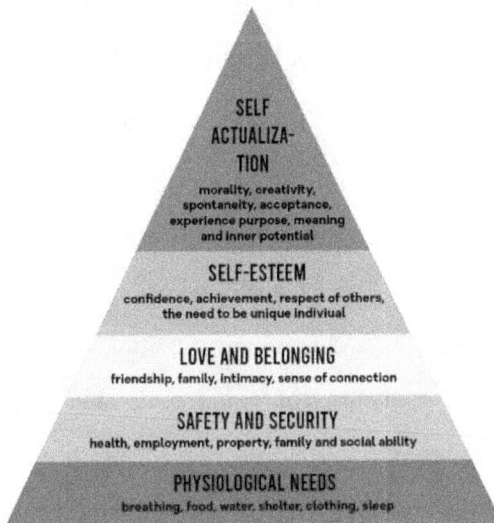

SELF ACTUALIZA-TION
morality, creativity, spontaneity, acceptance, experience purpose, meaning and inner potential

SELF-ESTEEM
confidence, achievement, respect of others, the need to be unique indiviual

LOVE AND BELONGING
friendship, family, intimacy, sense of connection

SAFETY AND SECURITY
health, employment, property, family and social ability

PHYSIOLOGICAL NEEDS
breathing, food, water, shelter, clothing, sleep

Chapter 1: Nourishing the Body

"I am conscious of the way I live and do things every day that nourish my body. I eat well, I work out, I try to manage stress, I get a good sleep in, and together, that does wonders." – Ella Woodward

The Food

The statement "you are what you eat" is particularly true as the way we nourish ourselves can help us feel rejuvenated and energetic and help us be in a pleasant mood, as opposed to feeling dull, dry, and low in energy.

Your food is your fuel. When you are looking to revive your physical body, starting with an understanding of fueling yourself is essential. This will create the foundation on which all other parts of your physical revival are based (and subsequently the revival of your mind and spirit), a necessity to facilitate your growth into your excellence. As we further uncover all the aspects of your revival, the interconnectedness will become clear.

The foods we consume are supposed to provide our bodies with various nutrients. I want to focus on the three macronutrients, which must be a part of every diet: **carbohydrates**, **fats**, and **proteins**. These nutrients, which are obtained from various foods, need to be ingested in specific quantities to ensure the minimal healthy functioning of our bodies. If you are missing certain nutrients from your diet, your energy and overall health will suffer. As we uncover what those are, I urge you to take notes, have a more detailed look at your diet as it stands, and understand how a healthy, functional diet may look for you. I know for many of you, it will involve changing your eating habits, patterns, and behaviors. But this is the only way to create the solid template necessary to add years to your life and life to your years as you grow into your excellence. This is the starting point of your growth.

Macronutrient #1: Carbohydrates

The most abundant sources of carbohydrates in our food are found in sugar, starch, and fiber. It is from here that carbohydrates are further subdivided into two categories: **simple** carbohydrates and **complex** carbohydrates. Simple carbohydrates are simple sugars. These are usually refined sugars that are found in many prepared foods, such as cereals and drinks. However, they can also be naturally occurring in fruits and milk products. The simple sugars that occur in foods in their natural or whole state are a healthier option (compared to the refined version) to consume and may also contain other vitamins and minerals.

Complex carbohydrates include starches and grain products. Some are better food choices than others. White flour, white rice, etc., have been processed and have lost much of their nutritional value and fiber, while unrefined grains still contain their vitamins, minerals, and fiber. Unrefined grains, such as brown rice and bulgar wheat, are healthier options. Additionally, they are rich in fiber, which facilitates the optimal functioning of our digestive system. Fiber is also filling and helps you to feel satiated sooner and fuller for longer periods, thus reducing the tendency of overeating and weight gain, which can lead to modern diseases of obesity and diabetes (to name a few).

When addressing the carbohydrates in your diet, the best options to ensure you are giving yourself the nourishing foundation you need are whole, unrefined grains, fruits, and vegetables. The daily recommendation for fruit and vegetable intake is about four hundred grams per day or five servings of 80 grams. A piece of fruit the size of a tennis ball or two cups of diced fruits would account for your fruit requirement, and 2 to 2-1/2 cups of vegetables per day is a useful, workable guide. It is advisable to consume your fruit first thing in the morning after a glass of warm water on an empty stomach. Some fruits, such as citrus, may increase acid production. Fiber and fructose in fruits may slow down the digestive system if eaten on an empty stomach, and for this reason, guava and oranges should not be consumed in the early mornings. It is unwise to consume your fruit after a meal as it may not be properly digested, and the nutrients may not be properly absorbed. At least 30 minutes should be allowed to elapse between a meal and your consumption of fruits. The myth that eating fruit at night allows you to add on weight is just that, a myth. However, if you consume a calorie-rich fruit like a banana every night after you have completed your calorie requirement for the day, you will add a few pounds by the end of the month. Raw vegetables or a salad should not be consumed on an empty stomach. They contain coarse fiber, which may increase the work burden on an empty stomach and may lead to flatulence and abdominal pains. There are no digestive benefits in eating your vegetables before, during, or after a meal. Vegetables can be eaten anytime, even as a late-night snack.

Macronutrient #2: Fats

Fats are an important part of our diets. Fats are an integral part of our physical makeup, along with muscle tissue and blood. It plays specific roles in the body. Having fat on your body is natural and only becomes a problem when certain types of fats are held in excess. There are two types of fat that your body produces: brown fat and white fat. Brown fat helps keep the body warm and is stored in tiny fat droplets. Brown fat is either constitutive (you were born with it, usually showing on adults around the neck and shoulders) or it is recruitable, meaning white fat can be converted to brown fat under appropriate conditions such as cooling your body down (e.g., with an ice bath, stepping out in cold weather or turning the thermostat in your homes down to about 66°F or 19°C.)

When we consume in excess, the excess nourishment is converted into white fat, which is stored around our various organ systems and forms visceral fat. White fat is the more common variety of fat. White fat stores energy in large fat droplets, which accumulate around the body and surround our internal organs or viscera. White fat keeps you warm through the insulation of your internal organs. White fat leads to obesity, and if stored around your midsection, it increases the risk of developing the metabolic syndrome, which increases the risk of heart disease, diabetes, and stroke.

There are three major classes of fat: Saturated, Unsaturated, and Trans Fat. Fats are composed of two smaller molecules, glycerol, and fatty acids. A **saturated fat** is one in which the fatty acids are composed of single bonds. Saturated fats are solids at room temperature. A small portion of saturated fats is acceptable in your diet. It should comprise only 6% of your daily energy source. At this level, saturated fats can improve your good cholesterol level and change dangerous cholesterol into a more benign form. At higher proportions, the reverse is true. It leads to a buildup of bad cholesterol in our bodies with plaque formation and an increased risk of cardiovascular disease.

Sources of Saturated Fats

- Fatty cuts of red meat

- Fatty cuts of Pork and chicken

- chicken skin and lard

- Dairy foods (milk, butter, cheese, sour cream, ice cream

- Coconut oils, palm oil

- Fried foods

Fats can also be **unsaturated**. These are liquids at room temperature and are the healthier, more beneficial variety. These unsaturated fats improve blood cholesterol levels, reduce inflammation, and stabilize heart rhythms. Unsaturated fats have a predominantly plant-based origin. They include vegetable oils, nuts, and seeds.

Unsaturated fats can be sub-divided into three sub-types:

1. Monounsaturated fats are in high concentrations in olives, peanut and canola oils, avocados, almonds, hazelnuts, pecans, pumpkin, and sesame seeds.

2. Polyunsaturated fats are found in high concentrations in sunflower, corn, soybean, flaxseed oils, walnuts, flaxseeds, fish, and canola oil.

3. Omega-3 fats are polyunsaturated and are obtained from our diets by eating fish 2-3 times per week. Omega -3 can also be had from flaxseeds, walnuts, canola, and soybean oil.

The higher the blood content of omega-3 fats, the healthier. Omega-3 fats reduce chronic inflammation in our bodies and lower the risk of premature death among older adults. The evidence suggests that if up to 15% of our daily calories come from polyunsaturated fats, we will have a reduced risk of heart disease. Recently we have learnt that replacing a carbohydrate-rich diet with one rich in unsaturated fats lowers blood pressure, improves lipid levels, and reduces cardiovascular risk. Coconut oil is particularly rich in saturated fat, containing a larger proportion of saturated fat than a fatty bit of beef. However, coconut oil tends to increase good cholesterol, and therefore, it is a saturated fat with a difference.

Trans Fats are produced through an industrial process (i.e., they are not naturally occurring). Hydrogen is added to vegetable oil, which then causes the oil to become solid at room temperature, hence the name "partially hydrogenated oil."

Sources of trans fats include:

- Baked goods such as cakes, cookies, and pies.

- Shortening

- Microwave popcorn.

- Frozen pizza

- Refrigerated dough, such as biscuits and rolls.

- Fried foods, including French fries, doughnuts, and fried chicken.

- Non-Dairy coffee creamer

- Stick margarine.

The reason restaurants will prefer to use this kind of oil for frying is because of its longer shelf life, so the oil does not have to be changed as often. Unfortunately, trans fats are the worst kinds of fats you can consume. Trans Fats raise your bad cholesterol levels while lowering your good cholesterol levels. A diet heavy in trans fats increases the risk of heart disease, which is the leading cause of death in adults. To keep your body in good health, a prerequisite for growing into your excellence, be mindful of your consumption of fast food or fried foods and the trans fats to which you are exposed and will be ingesting. Consuming trans fats is a sure ticket to poor health and challenges your cardiovascular health.

Macronutrient #3: Proteins

Proteins are the third essential macronutrient you require to nourish your physical body. Amino acids are the building blocks of Proteins and are essential components of all living things. There are three types of proteins, each playing a specific role in your body. I will highlight these features.

Fibrous proteins include keratin and collagen and form part of the connective tissues in the body, such as tendons, bones, and muscles. Therefore, they are necessary for facilitating support and movement. **Globular proteins** may function as enzymes, hormones, transport molecules, and even part of the body's defense system. These types of proteins are integrally involved in the normal functioning of our bodies. The third major type of protein is **membrane proteins**. These are in the cell membrane and perform a variety of functions. For example, these proteins may help transport substances across the cell membranes or serve as receptors on which substances can bind and bring about changes within the cell. This is just a glimpse of all the functions of proteins, and as you can see, it goes far beyond just building muscle!

There is a vast array of foods that function as protein sources that are available to us, including:

- lean meat, poultry, fish

- eggs

- dairy products (such as cottage cheese and yogurt)

- seeds and nuts

- beans, legumes (lentils) and soya products

About 12-20% of your daily calories should come from protein. Your body stores excess protein as fat. Excess amino acids are transported in the bloodstream to the liver, where they are used to create new proteins.

Beyond the essential *macro*nutrients of carbohydrates, fat, and protein, your body also requires an array of *micro*nutrients. These include dietary fiber, minerals, vitamins, and water. Every nutrient plays its role when it comes to bringing more vitality to your physical body. Starting with understanding the macronutrients and how they are part of your diet, it is the essential starting point to revive your body, as we aim to provide you with the tools you need to grow into your excellence. When the carbs, fats, and proteins are balanced in your diet, you will feel more energized, and you will begin to function at a higher level physically. 20-35% of your total daily calories should come from fat; this means eating 50 to 80 grams of fat per day. Carbohydrates, on the other hand, should comprise 45-65% of your total daily calories, and 10-30 percent of your daily calories should be made up of proteins.

Reflection:

Am I aware of what I eat, or do I just eat whatever, whenever? How does it make me feel?

Do I eat a good balance of complex carbs and simple carbs?

Do I eat enough healthy fats?

What are the main sources of protein in my diet?

_____

_____

_____

_____

_____

_____

In the next chapter, I want to give you a snapshot of the basic dietary patterns we follow (omnivore, vegetarian, and vegan), and examine the benefits of them all. So, you can begin reflecting on which may suit you best. Again, meeting your physiological needs first will set you up for success as you grow into excellence.

Chapter 2: Source of Food

"Want to learn to eat a lot? Here it is eat a little. That way you will be around long enough to eat a lot." – Tony Robbins

Types of Food

Human beings are **omnivores** in that they consume both plant and animal products. **Carnivores** main source of nourishment are animal products, and **herbivores** main source of nourishment are plant-based products. I am sure many of you are asking and wondering which is the best choice when thinking about how to revive your physical body. Let us examine both: a diet that is more animal product-based and one that is more plant-based. There are certainly benefits with the use of each, but the question remains: which is healthier overall? Remember, we are preparing you to grow into your excellence.

I find it fascinating that biblical scholars have rushed to suggest that human beings were never intended to eat animals' flesh but were granted permission by God because of the lack of vegetation after the great flood in the story of Noah. (These examples are in the book of Genesis.) Other stories found in the bible also show examples of the life span of men being greatly reduced by hundreds of years, generation after generation, thus further presenting an observation that the human life span has been reduced with the introduction of animal-based products to his/her diet. In today's modern world, which diet is healthier? I hear you ask. As we explore these diets, we are trying to create a solid and vibrant foundation on which to build, so you can grow into excellence.

Carnivore Diet

Supporters of an animal product-based diet believe that meat should be an integral part of your diet. It has various nutrients. It is a source of complete high-quality protein, iron, and vitamin B12. Meat products in our diet are highly beneficial. Studies have shown that a high-protein diet, which includes ingesting meat, can increase our metabolism, reduce hunger, and help us feel fuller for longer. (Of course, this can then be associated with weight loss.) Additionally, having a diet high in animal protein may also help you retain muscle mass, strengthen bones, and maintain ideal levels of iron in your body. The main benefit of including meat in our diet is that it provides a source of protein.

A snapshot of the benefits of having meat in your diet includes:

- Strengthen bones and aid iron absorption!

- A source of complete amino acids, thus helping to build muscle mass.

- It strengthens your immune system through the production of antibodies.

- It contains a full spectrum of micronutrients and vitamins that can promote a healthier state of being.

If having a diet that includes meat products contributes to your health, why is it that there has been a steady decline in the life span of human beings since the introduction of meat to our diets?

Multiple studies from Oxford University found that there was an 11% reduced risk of cancer among vegetarians and a 19% reduced risk of cancer among vegans. The incidence of some types of cancers is higher in countries with a large intake of red meat. Hungary and Uruguay had the highest overall rate of cancer in 2020. These countries, including Argentina, have among the world's largest red and processed meat consumption in the world. Conversely, India and South Asia are among the countries in the world with the lowest per capita red meat consumption. Interestingly, India and South Asia countries have among the lowest incidence of bowel cancers. Another interesting observation among these countries with the lowest incidence of bowel cancers, their diet is heavily plant-based.

We are providing you with the necessary tools to allow you to add years to your life and life to your years as you grow into your excellence. In that case, we recommend that you avoid exposure to factors that increase your risk of developing certain diseases. Could a diet that includes meat products be a contributing factor to illnesses that affect the general population? Would it be best to recommend a plant-based diet as the superior choice? Since we started consuming meat regularly, there has been a clear increase in heart disease, cancers, strokes, diabetes, obesity, elevated cholesterol levels, acne, and, for men, erectile dysfunction that affects our health year after year. This causes a reduction in our overall health and life span.

Let us now explore the virtues of a plant-based diet and all it may offer. We must be familiar with both diet types, an integral step, when growing into excellence. As Maslow cautioned in his hierarchy of needs, physiological needs must be addressed for self-actualization to be achieved.

Beef and other Red Processed Meats

Red meat (any meat that is dark red in color before cooked), which includes veal, pork, lamb, beef, and goat meat does have health benefits but meat consumption has been linked to many health challenges. Research reported in the International Journal of Epidemiology in 2019 concluded that even moderate meat-eating increases bowel cancer risk.

Processed meat is meat that is not sold fresh but instead has been cured, salted, smoked, or otherwise preserved, so bacon, sausages, hot dogs, salami, and pepperoni would be included in this category. White meats like fresh turkey, chicken, and fish do not appear to increase your risk of bowel cancer.

Three chemicals from red and processed meats have been identified as possible triggers in the development of cancer. These include (a) haem (the red pigment found mostly in red meat), (b) nitrates and nitrites (used to keep processed meats fresher for longer), and heterocyclic amines and polycyclic amines (this is produced when meat is cooked at an elevated temperature). All three compounds can damage the cells in our bowels, and it is the accumulation of this damage over time that increases cancer risk.

Data analyzed from half a million UK adults over almost seven years found that moderately processed and red meat eaters, those consuming on average seventy-nine grams per day, had a 32% increased risk of bowel cancer compared to people eating less than 11 grams of red and processed meat daily.

Eating red processed meats increases your risk of developing bowel cancer. People who eat more than 90 grams of cooked red and processed meat a day are advised to reduce this amount to 70 grams or less to try to reduce the risk of developing bowel cancer.

Although admittedly, there are benefits to the consumption of red and processed meats, the evidence indicates that there is a risk of developing cancer from prolonged use of more than 79 grams daily. The consumption of large portions of red meat daily will increase your risk of bowel cancer, which is reported to be on the rise among the younger age groups.

Types of Plant-Based Diets

There are a variety of plant-based diets and to distinguish them we need to look at what is included and excluded from the diet.

Lacto Ovo Vegetarian Diet: One of the most popular plant-based diets. As indicated, no meat (beef, pork, poultry, fish, etc.) is consumed in this diet. Though dairy products such as cheese and yogurt as well as eggs are used.

Ovo Vegetarian Diet: This diet type excludes all meats and dairy products. Only eggs and plant-based dishes are included.

Pescatarian Diet: In this diet, there is no dairy, eggs, beef, chicken, or poultry consumed. Only fish and plant-based dishes are used.

Vegan Diet: Rising in popularity, a vegan diet excludes animal-based products in any form. Plant-based dishes are the only foods consumed in this diet.

Virtues of a Vegetarian Diet

Now presented with the diverse types of vegetarian diets, you are probably wondering which one is the healthiest for your body. What should you include in your diet, and which foods should you exclude in the long term? Internationally, the vegetarian diet has health benefits, including lower incidences of heart disease, cancer, and type 2 diabetes. Let us examine key elements of a vegetarian diet that can boost your health.

Inflammation

Studies have indicated an association between degenerative diseases and chronic inflammation. Where does this inflammation in the body stem from, and how can we control it? Firstly, inflammation is a naturally occurring process in the body, but it is of two types: acute and chronic inflammation. Our tissues can become inflamed when dealing with an injury, and this is a necessary component of the healing process. Short-term (acute) inflammation differs from chronic inflammation, which is associated with diseases, such as cancers, arterial plaque formation, heart attacks, strokes, diabetes, and autoimmune diseases such as type 1 diabetes and Systemic lupus erythematosus. Free radicals trigger chronic inflammation. Free radicals are high-energy particles derived from essential metabolic processes in the human body. They can cause significant disruption to many physiological processes. This type of inflammation is seen most often in diets laden with animal products.

When your body is injured, it will naturally react with inflammation to heal itself. This type of inflammation, acute inflammation, which occurs, for example, after a bruise or a cut, is a healthy, natural process.

Studies have shown that eating meat, cheese, and highly processed foods is associated with elevated levels of chronic inflammation in our bodies. This type of inflammation, chronic inflammation, is a dangerous type of inflammation that is associated with many chronic diseases. Therefore, it makes good sense to have a plant-based diet, rich in fruits and vegetables, to stave off chronic inflammation in your body and give yourself the best opportunity to ward off chronic conditions and diseases.

Microbiome

In our bodies live trillions of microorganisms, which collectively are known as the microbiome. These microorganisms, while you cannot see them, are crucial to our overall health. They help in the digestion of our foods, produce essential nutrients, contribute to our immune system, keep our gut tissues healthy, and help to protect against cancer. They also reduce the risk of obesity, diabetes, vascular disease, autoimmune disease, inflammatory bowel disease, and liver disease.

These healthy microorganisms and bacteria feed on the fiber found in a variety of fruits and vegetables. Plant-based meals promote the growth of gut-friendly bacteria. Consuming meals high in dairy, eggs, and meat products will encourage the growth of disease-promoting bacteria. These bacteria can lead to diseases, as listed above.

There is an increased production of Trimethylamine N-oxide (TMAO) found in the bloodstream after consuming animal products. Consuming the chemicals choline or carnitine, which is found in meats, poultry, eggs, seafood, and dairy, causes the gut bacteria to make Trimethylamine (TMA), which is converted by the liver to Trimethylamine N-oxide (TMAO). It is alarming to note that studies have shown that people with elevated levels of TMAO in their blood have more than twice the risk of heart attacks, strokes, and serious cardiovascular problems compared with people who have lower levels. High TMAO in the blood will lead to chronic kidney disease, increased risk of Type 2 diabetes, and worsening levels of cholesterol plaque in our vascular system (leading to a higher risk of heart disease and stroke).

It is not hard to draw conclusions then, is it?... When you consume a plant-based diet, you will make little to no TMAO because of your healthier gut microbiome. The benefits of a plant-based diet are quick as it takes only a few days for the gut bacterial flora to change. How exciting to know that making a few changes today can make huge improvements to your gut health and influence your overall health!

The Best Self-caring Diet

I am sure it is now becoming clear that a diet based solely on plants is optimal for your health! This is referred to as a **vegan diet**. Vegan diets are abundant in vitamins B1, C, and E, as well as folic acid, magnesium, and iron. An additional benefit is the diet is low in cholesterol and saturated fats. Should one be concerned if you are asked to avoid foods that hitherto were part of your regular diet? One of the major concerns when going vegan is an increased risk of vitamin B12 deficiency, but it can be remedied through the consumption of fortified plant-based food or a vitamin B12 supplement. (The recommended daily dietary allowance for Vitamin B12 is only 1.8 micrograms for children and adults, 2.4 micrograms for pregnant women, and 2.8 micrograms for breastfeeding women.) Be mindful as well that there are several factors that can affect the absorption of vitamin B12, such as age, antacids, and the drug metformin (commonly used to treat type 2 diabetes).

There are many resources that lead to a healthy and balanced vegan diet. When using vegan diets, you reap all the benefits we have been discussing, but also increase your intake of beneficial antioxidants. Antioxidants optimize how your cells repair damaged DNA and can slow down the ageing process of your cells, which can lead to a more dynamic and longer life as well as facilitate your growth into your excellence!

To fulfill the world population's demand for food, genetically modified organisms (GMOs) were developed to help increase the yields of crops. However, studies now show that GMO-exposed foods can lead to a multitude of health complications, such as hepatic, pancreatic, renal, and reproductive harmful effects. Knowing this now, I highly recommend that you choose to consume non-GMO foods as much as possible. Another excellent choice is choosing whole foods or foods that are as close to their original state as possible. Even if foods are labeled vegan, they can be highly processed and can be unhealthy. Be mindful and remember, you are what you eat.

My Personal Experience

I recognize that it is easier said than done. Truly, after eating meat products all your life and now recognizing the virtues of a vegan diet, deciding to optimize your health to facilitate a longer, healthier life as well as a more vivacious life is not easy.

For me, I grew up observing the preparation of meat dishes, smelling the enticing aroma of such dishes being prepared, and enjoying the prepared dishes, often craving more. Still, as I started learning more and more about the virtues of veganism, it became apparent to me that I had to make a change if I wanted to add years to my life and life to my years.

The transition was not easy, with starts and stops along the way. Motivated by the adage that by the yard it is hard, but by the inch, everything is a cinch, I tried. I dropped red meats from my diet, only using chicken and fish dishes with the occasional relapse to enjoy an ox-tail dish. During the process, I had the opportunity to have a doppler scan on my common carotid arteries, which carries blood to the head, neck, and face. The results were not pretty, with arterial plaques seen in both arteries, thereby informing me of the risks of having a stroke. When I questioned how the process could be slowed or reversed, the answer was simple: change to a vegan diet. This was a major light bulb moment; was I prepared to keep doing what I had always done while I slowly but progressively marched to a disabled life or maybe worse? Was it time to sacrifice the toxins of my ordinary meat-eating life and claim an opportunity to feed myself the healthier option of a vegan diet? And in so doing, give myself the foundation for adding years to my life and life to my years? My father, a meat eater, died at age 81, his mother a vegan, died at age 115. For me, there was no doubt in my choice since my focus was on the addition of years to my life and life to my years while growing into my excellence.

I started preparing my own meals, which were bulgar wheat and lentils. Initially, the taste was repulsive, but with experience and a few tweaks, it became an enjoyable dish. My salads were uncooked vegetable matter. To add to the attractiveness of the dish, I combined the grated green cabbage with the purple, maroon ones and doused the grated cabbages with colorless apple cider vinegar. I enjoyed this for a while and gradually learnt to prepare other dishes. If there is a need for milk in my drinks, I use almond milk. If there is a need for sugar, which is rare, I use stevia.

Since going full-time on my vegan-based meals, the lassitude and need for caffeinated beverages have disappeared. I am experiencing a level of clarity of my thoughts, which reminds me of when I was in my twenties. My mood rarely fluctuates, being always pleasant and friendly. My drive for physical activity has also risen. My bowels are a lot more regular; I have less problem with my weight control, and overall, I feel more like the self that I consider ideal! I am grateful I am now focusing on a vegan diet, and I love the way it makes me feel.

Hydration

Human beings are composed of at least 65% water. This fact alone should make you understand the importance of drinking enough water throughout the day. You need to make hydration a priority. The reasons we need water and how it affects our bodies are extensive! I'll touch on several key points to get you motivated.

Firstly, you are asking yourself what volume of water you need to drink to be properly hydrated on any regular day. Health professionals suggest adults should aim for a *minimum* of two liters (approx. 68 oz) a day. To make it easy to remember just follow the 8 x 8 principle: have an 8oz glass of water eight times a day. If you have trouble keeping track of the volume of water you have drunk throughout the day, I recommend that you drink all your water out of one water bottle. Know how many bottles you need to drink by the end of the day to receive your minimum hydration and keep track of how many times you fill your bottle. (An easy hydration hack!)

The body's response to hydration varies in symptoms and severity. When inadequately hydrated, there can be an imbalance in your blood sugar levels. You may experience headaches or even have a change in your mood. Other symptoms may manifest as fatigue, mental slowness, irritability, and a rise in your temperature. All your physiological processes need an adequate amount of water.

Externally, hydration gives your skin a healthy glow and can reduce the appearance of wrinkles. Water lubricates joints and helps with the delivery of oxygen to our tissues. It also helps in the production of mucus, saliva, and digestive juices. Did you know that water helps in cushioning your brain and spinal cord as well as other sensitive body structures? Hydration keeps these precious organs healthy and free from traumatic physical damage. Water is essential to perspiring (your sweat is

90% water!), which not only helps regulate body temperature (even when you are not working out) but also aids in excreting toxins from the body.

There is a correlation between hydration and weight management. Water can act as an appetite suppressant and seems to allow our bodies to use up more calories in our resting state. In animal studies, water was shown to have a fat-burning capacity. If you are trying to manage your weight, staying adequately hydrated is important.

Can you consume too much water? The answer is yes. In a healthy person, that would be extremely hard to do. Your kidneys are responsible for eliminating water from your body and can eliminate 0.8 to 1L of fluid every hour. You may run into problems when you drink *more* than a liter of water every hour. Excessive water in our system causes a diluted amount of sodium in our body, which can then lead to an excess of fluid being absorbed into our cells and results in swelling. Obviously, taking the body out of this homeostasis (balanced) state can be harmful to your health. Consuming the ideal 2L/day will not only make you feel better physically, but it also leads to positive outcomes for your mind and spirit. You will *feel* better by drinking more water! This is an inexpensive and quick solution for a variety of ailments.

Reflection:

What kind of diet am I currently consuming?

Why would I consider switching to a plant-based diet?

Are there any benefits to me in switching to a plant-based diet?

What will it take for me to switch to a plant-based diet?

Am I willing to switch to a plant based or vegan diet?

What are my favorite fruits and vegetables?

What is my average daily water consumption?

Have I noticed a correlation with what I eat and how I feel physically (Does the food I eat contribute to aches I feel or digestive issues etc.?)

_____

_____

_____

_____

_____

_____

_____

_____

_____

Of course, I am going to encourage you to grab a glass of water and continue reading on while we continue exploring how we can elevate your health to create a solid foundation for your revival and to facilitate the growth into your excellence. Let us look at elements around us and how they impact us, specifically air and sunlight.

Chapter 3: Nutrition versus Nourishment

The Difference

On the surface, both nutrition and nourishment appear to mean the same thing, but let us take a closer look. Nutrition is the study of food and how it affects the health and growth of the body. The foods have nutrients that contribute to the growth and well-being of our bodies. The obvious question, then, is how does nutrition differ from nourishment? Nourishment for our bodies provides our body with the food that is necessary for life, growth, and good health.

Immediately, nutrition differs from nourishment in one key area; whereas nutrition contributes to the growth and well-being of our body, Nourishment goes further by ensuring good health of our bodies. Nutrition can define anything in our diet. It is the items we ingest to keep us satiated, and it may or may not be healthy. We know that all the food we consume may not be healthy and may not be good for us. When we seek to be nourished, we aim for the consumption of foods that will both keep us satisfied and will also help to keep our bodies healthy.

Proteins, Fats, and Carbohydrates: Nutrition, not necessarily Nourishment

From the above, one must admit that nutrition and nourishment are not identical. Nutrition is a grade of nourishment, with different foods and the methods of preparation varying in the degree of nourishment that they can provide. Foods vary in their ability to nourish our bodies. It is not how much we consume; it is the quality of the foods to which we are exposed. Fast food may not be nourishing, but it plays a role in satisfying hunger. Fast food is nutrition, not nourishment. The oil in which these foods are prepared exposes the consumer to a high dose of trans fats, which add to the taste of the food but fail to adequately nourish our bodies. Obviously, fried chicken and or chips provide proteins and carbohydrates, which comprise macronutrients that our body needs to function, but continuous exposure to these foods is damaging to our general health and, more precisely, to our cardiovascular health.

Foods we eat do vary in their ability to nourish our bodies. To that end, we appreciate that foods are not equally nutritious. They may have components that contribute to aspects of our well-being, but over time, they are toxic to our bodies. We must be wise in choosing the foods or intake which will make the best contribution to our health. Above, we mentioned fast food, specifically fried chicken, as not being nourishment because of the trans fats. Suppose the chicken was prepared differently, say the skin was removed, and the chicken was either boiled or baked. This would improve the nourishment potential of the chicken to our bodies. It is not only the food that determines its degree of nourishment to our bodies but the manner in which it is prepared. Fried foods are not as nourishing as the same food boiled or baked.

What about smoked meats? I hear you ask. The National Cancer Institute warns that smoked foods present both Heterocyclic Amines (HCA) and Polycyclic Aromatic Hydrocarbons (PAH) to our bodies, which are mutagenic – they increase the risk of DNA damage. High exposure to these compounds increases the risk of intestinal tract cancers. Thus, although the taste of these foods is delightful, their nourishing ability cannot be commended. Similarly, cured meats such as sausages and cooked ham, bacon, and bologna, although enjoyable to some, are found to have an almost direct relationship as a causative agent for bowel cancers. In populations in which there is a high consumption of cured meats, the incidence of bowel cancer is among the highest in the world. Knowing this, we need to be more selective in the foods we choose to consume as we grow into excellence.

Similarly, diets high in refined starches, such as white flour, pastries, cookies, muffins, cakes, waffles, pancakes, pretzels, pizza dough, and white rice, contribute to a higher risk of diabetes, heart disease, and weight gain. Again, although these food substances provide a macronutrient, which is carbohydrates, they would not be highly nourishing foods. Potatoes are refined grains because of their carbohydrate content and behave similar to refined starches. Although carbohydrates are our body's preferred source of energy, refined carbohydrates have fewer nutrients than wholegrain ones and so are less nourishing.

Excessive dietary intake of fats leads to obesity, coronary heart disease, and certain types of cancer. High consumption of saturated -fatty acids is a risk factor for cardiovascular disease. Fats, though a macronutrient, are not nourishing to our bodies and, in excess, can cause significant disease. We must be careful with what we eat to ensure we are able to grow into excellence.

Micronutrients

These are nutritional elements, vitamins, and minerals needed by the body in tiny amounts. Their impact on the body's health is critical, and deficiency in any of them can cause severe and life-threatening conditions. Functions of these micronutrients include the production of hormones, enzymes, and other substances needed for growth and development. Deficiencies in iron, vitamin A, and iodine are among the most common worldwide. The effects of the deficiency in pregnant ladies and children are most frequently noted. Deficiencies can cause visible and dangerous health conditions but can also lead to less clinically notable reductions in energy level, mental capacity, and clarity. They either occur naturally or are added to various foods to improve their ability to nourish our bodies.

For optimal nourishment, one must try to ensure access to wholesome foods, prepared with the utmost care, and in cases where nutrients may be absent, seek out supplements to ensure optimal care of your body to facilitate your growth into excellence.

Water

We have extolled the health benefits of water. But like chicken, additives to water can prove damaging to our health. Communities around the world have chlorine added to their supply of drinking water, the reason advanced for this practice is to enhance the purity of the water. Chlorine acts as an antiseptic and serves to keep the water piped into our homes free of dangerous microbes. Research indicates that no community that had its water so treated has a low incidence of cardiovascular disease.

You may wonder, is there a causal link? Every high school chemistry student learns that chlorine occupies one of the top positions in the electrochemical series (a table of substances in order of their oxidizing abilities, the strongest oxidizing agents occupying the top of the table). Chlorine occupies one of the top positions in this table, testifying to its potency as an oxidizing agent. The link though may still not be immediately obvious. Allow me to explain.

Contrary to the bad name given to cholesterol, our body produces about 75% to 90% of its cholesterol needs in the liver, and only about 10% to 25% of our total cholesterol comes from our foods. Yet the attack on cholesterol by the establishment immediately brings you to the conclusion that something is amiss. Why is our body working as hard to poison itself? 75% to 90% of this poison is synthesized by our body. Obviously, there must be a role for this heavily produced substance in our body, and it may not be as dangerous as feared. Cholesterol is important for a variety of processes in our body. It is integral in the formation of the cell membrane and its repair. There are an average of thirty trillion human cells in our body, and everyone contains a cell membrane that surrounds the cell and separates it from its neighbor. Therefore, there is a need for significant amounts of cholesterol, but that is not all. Cholesterol plays a vital role in the production of the sex hormones: estrogen, progesterone, and testosterone, as well as the stress hormone cortisol. Our body therefore needs substantial amounts of cholesterol, hence the production in our liver. There are two basic types of cholesterol, (a) Good cholesterol, or high-density lipoprotein (HDL) [this type of cholesterol is involved in the transportation of LDL to the liver and from here it is excreted from the body, hence its sobriquet, "good cholesterol" and bad cholesterol or low-density lipoprotein (LDL). The bulk of the cholesterol produced by our bodies is of the LDL variety. So, again it begs the question, why is the body producing large amounts of this bad substance? Is LDL really bad? Could it be transformed LDL that causes it to get a bad name? How does this relate to chlorine, you ask?

Chlorine in Our Water Supply

Chlorine is among the most potent oxidizing agents known to man. An oxidizing agent works by oxidizing substances. LDL is not bad, but it can undergo oxidation to give rise to a variety called oxidized LDL. This oxidized variety is the type of LDL that is deadly to our cardiovascular system. Oxidized LDL is smaller and stickier than the parent LDL. The oxidized LDL, because of its stickiness, adheres to the walls of our blood vessels. Calcium, with time, sticks to this oxidized LDL, giving rise to plaque formation and narrowing the affected blood vessel. Not only that, but the oxidized LDL is atherosclerotic, meaning it induces inflammatory changes in our blood vessels, which leads to the progressive narrowing of the affected vessel. If the plaque so formed is unstable, bits can break off and travel elsewhere in the blood. When it gets to a vessel through which it is unable to pass, it simply blocks that vessel, cutting off the flow of blood distal to the occlusion with devastating consequences. In the brain, it leads to a stroke. In the lungs, it leads to a pulmonary embolus, which can be deadly, and in the heart, it leads to a heart attack. If it occurs in a limb, the portion of the limb distal to the occlusion dies and may have devastating consequences for the affected limb and individual.

This is a synopsis of the association between the chlorine in our drinking water and cardiovascular disease. Even our drinking water may fail to adequately nourish our bodies. Chlorine is not only present in our tap water but also brought to our homes in the bottled water we buy from the food stores. In the United Kingdom, the amount of chlorine in our tap water is 0.5 milligrams per liter or less. Shopping around the supermarkets for bottled water is disappointing because they all have varying amounts of chlorine. One suggestion is to boil your water to get rid of much of its chlorine content.

Reflection:

How does nutrition differ from nourishment?

Would a diet of only fried chicken be nourishing?

Is there any other component that needs to be in food apart from the macronutrients of carbohydrates, fats, and proteins to ensure that the food is nourishing?

Is fried food more nourishing than baked foods?

Is there any relationship between tap water and cardiovascular disease?

Do micronutrients play a role in our nourishment?

What percentage of cholesterol does our body produce?

Which variety of cholesterol is dangerous?

Are red and processed meats nourishing?

_____

_____

_____

_____

_____

_____

_____

_____

Chapter 4: Our Environment

"Although our bodies are bounded with skin, and we can differentiate between outside and inside, they cannot exist except in a certain kind of natural environment." – Alan Watts

The Environmental Challenges

To say that we do not live in a vacuum is certainly stating the obvious! As we go about our "day-to-day" activities, there is no denying that the environment around us profoundly impacts our physical bodies, both positively and negatively. To stay in line with our goal of adding years to your life and life to your years, as you grow into your excellence, it is worth taking some time to investigate some major aspects of your environment, reflect on how they are affecting you now and how you can make some changes in order to harness the most positive aspects of both the **air** and **sunlight** that surrounds you.

Air

When you think of your relationship to air, you may think solely of the oxygen that we need. air only comprises about 21% of the volume of air surrounding us. The air forms a blanket that acts as a sort of environmental shield for our bodies. It maintains temperature by trapping heat from the sun (this regulated temperature is vital for our bodies), and it protects our bodies from the harmful effects of ultraviolet radiation from the sun.

The ozone layer, a part of the earth's atmosphere, is integrally involved in shielding us from the harmful effects of ultraviolet radiation. This complex process involves absorbing the bulk of ultraviolet radiation from the sun. Air is the medium through which the carbon dioxide we exhale is transported. Carbon dioxide is used by plants in photosynthesis to produce food, and in return, the plants give off oxygen, which we use for our own needs through respiration.

Clean air helps improve your blood pressure and heart rate and facilitates your digestion. Clean air strengthens your immune system and clears your lungs. Exposure to fresh air leads to an elevation in mood, energy levels, and a sharper mind. Breathing is automatic; putting the focus on the quality of air we breathe is imperative. Particulate matter in air of 2.5 microns or smaller presents many health challenges. The smaller the particles, the greater the health challenge. Particles less than 10 microns in diameter can get deep into your lungs and may even enter the bloodstream. Epidemiological and toxicological studies view ambient fine particulate ($PM_{2.5}$) as particles having an aerodynamic diameter of less than 2.5 microns, as a significant danger to human health. Particles of this size are mostly absorbed through our respiratory system, where they can pass through our air sacs and reach our bloodstream. Recent data indicates that fine particulate matter, or $PM_{2.5}$ is responsible for nearly 4 million deaths globally from a range of illnesses. These illnesses include cardiopulmonary illnesses, such as heart disease, respiratory infections, chronic lung disease, cancers, preterm births, and other illnesses.

You may be wondering whether you should try to measure this particulate matter to determine your clean air safety zones. We are not asking you to do so; we are just sharing useful information to facilitate your health as you grow into excellence. Particulate matter is made of solid and liquid particles that are discharged into the air from exhaust fumes, burning bush, industrial activity, and smoking.

The World Health Organization reported that around 7 million people die every year due to exposure to polluted air. In 2016, there were 4.2 million deaths in low/middle-income countries. Air pollution is caused by a mixture of substances such as gases, particles, and biological components in the earth's atmosphere. The toxic effects caused by particle pollution on humans are dependent on their size, surface area, and chemical composition. Air pollution is the single largest causative agent of various diseases. This is most clearly seen in elderly people, particularly in those with preexisting cardiopulmonary diseases. The sizes of the particulate matter causing air pollution are described as $PM_{0.1}$ called ultrafine particles, $PM_{2.5}$ called fine particles, refers to particles, which are 2.5 micrometers or less in diameter. PM_{10} describes particles less than or equal to 10 micrometers in diameter. $PM_{2.5}$ is characterized by fine particles that have a large surface area, and they are better able to accumulate than the PM_{10} particles. They also remain suspended in the air for longer periods and are more likely to be inhaled.

We require clean air to live optimally. Living in more urban areas where the air quality may not be brilliant, taking a walk in the early morning hours when the air quality is better would be highly recommended. If you live in a more rural setting where there is less pollution, getting outside daily, preferably in the morning for a 30-minute walk, is rewarding. When outside during your walks, focus on your breathing and take deeper breaths than usual. This will aid in the fresh air entering deep into your lungs and helping deliver all its benefits to your body. Having a daily dose of clean air will make a great impact on your revival, contributing years to your life, and the act of walking will contribute to your overall health! By choosing to walk in the morning, you will not only get cleaner, fresher air, but the act of walking will encourage the contraction and relaxation of your muscles and will lead to enhanced circulation.

Global warming and climate change are having a deleterious effect on many aspects of our life and health. Global warming has led to the buildup of greenhouse gases (such as carbon dioxide and methane) in the atmosphere, causing ambient temperatures to rise. Using fossil fuels for travel and the farming of animals are major contributors to the damage to our environment. Deforestation, which leads to fewer trees absorbing carbon dioxide and producing oxygen, is a recipe for ill health for us all in the time to come. If the temperature of ambient air on the planet continues to rise, it will make living conditions on Earth that much harsher and may eventually render the Earth uninhabitable. If we do not come together (citizens and leaders alike) and take full responsibility for this issue, our health and the well-being of future generations cannot be guaranteed.

I am sure you have read about how you can make a difference in addressing the issue of global warming. On a personal level, the choice of a plant-based diet will help to reduce the impact of global warming. Not only is a vegan diet beneficial to your body, as we discussed in the previous chapter, but it is also beneficial for the environment! You may not be aware, but creating less of a demand for animal products will affect the health of our planet. Animal farming is one of the greatest contributors to global warming. For example, take the production of beef and the inevitable production of methane gas. Methane gas is 80 times more damaging to the environment than carbon dioxide over a 20-year period. The non-consumption of beef and other animal products has a positive long-term benefit on the atmosphere. Choosing a plant-based diet is really a win-win solution when you look at it through this lens. Good for you and good for the environment of the planet!

Sometimes, you may not be able to see or feel the direct effects of what is contaminating the air around you. Great technological advances are certainly improving our lives in multiple ways by allowing great ease of communication, helping us to stay connected, and creating business opportunities. However, with the move to more online-based communication and the demand for it to be faster every year, comes an increase in various sources of electromagnetic radiation. This type of air pollution is one we cannot see or feel, but it is most certainly present and beyond our immediate control. We trust the scientific communities and governments to safeguard our interests and our health when it comes to this specific element in our environment. However, now that electromagnetic radiation is adversely affecting your environment and can affect your well-being, it is empowering as you can now advocate for your own health and safety with your political leaders.

Living in polluted cities and towns is part of living in this modern era. We cannot escape it, and it is something we must learn to navigate. Therefore, it is of utter importance that you remember each breath you take can impact your health. Getting out for early morning fresh air or taking steps to reduce the electromagnetic pollution in your home (i.e., turning off electronics when not in use and/or reducing their use altogether) is imperative for reviving your body. Acting for your health empowers you.

Sunlight

Your relationship to sunlight is an essential pillar in leading a healthy and active life. It is a natural part of our surroundings and environment, which we too often take for granted. One of the most popular benefits of exposing yourself to sunlight is an increase in your body's production of vitamin D. Our body's vitamin D production is triggered by the sun! Vitamin D is vital in combating chronic inflammation. It lowers blood pressure, improves brain function, and helps improve your mood. It helps strengthen bones and teeth as well. If you live in the northern hemisphere, it is strongly recommended that you take a Vitamin D supplement during the winter months when you are exposed to much less sunlight.

While we are talking about winter months with less sunlight, it is important to touch upon Seasonal Affective Disorder (SAD). SAD is a mood disorder where people manifest depressive symptoms during the winter months. There is a direct correlation between increased cases of SAD and reduced sunlight. Sunlight produces serotonin, a "feel-good hormone" in the body. A widely accepted treatment for SAD is light therapy. Light therapy is the exposure to an artificial light source that is not a source of UV light. The light enters through the eye and, in a sense, tricks the brain into thinking it is exposed to more natural daylight hours. The production of serotonin is triggered by light entering the eye, so even if you don't get any exposure to the sun itself, having a light box handy on your desk or at home can ensure that serotonin is produced, even without a daily dose of the sun or daylight. (Light boxes are readily available for purchase online or at wellness stores). Light therapy may prove to be an inexpensive way to naturally boost your mood, and, therefore, your overall wellness. I urge you to try it!

For your well-being, there are hazards to excessive exposure to the sun. Sun exposure can lead to skin damage, such as sunburn, premature skin ageing, and even cancer. (Frighteningly, 90% of skin cancers are induced by excessive exposure to the sun.) Avoiding direct sunlight, especially in the afternoon when the sun's ultraviolet light is most potent, is best. At all times, be mindful to stay covered and use appropriate sunscreen.

Reflection:

How often do I get out in the morning for fresh air?

How often do I go outside to gain the benefit of some sunlight?

Do I ever feel like I have a low mood in the winter months?

Does your mood in the winter months differ from the summer months?

_____

_____

_____

_____

_____

_____

I hope that you are feeling more inspired to get outside for some fresh air and sunlight and consider a plant-based diet. Our modern lives revolve around work and screen time. It is easy to forget about how such simple factors as clean air and a daily dose of sunlight are necessary to truly live our best possible life. There are more key aspects to the foundation one must create to gain vitality and add years to your life and life to your years. The final building blocks I want to discuss are being physically active, the importance of rest, and the necessity for temperance. It is always about keeping things in balance.

Chapter 5: Factors That Impact Your Body

"Nothing happens until something moves." – Albert Einstein

Controllable Factors

The final key to the revival of your body, as you prepare to grow into your excellence, is to control those things over which you have control. I want us to examine exercise, rest, and the practice of temperance. These are the final pieces when creating that solid foundation you need to continue your journey of adding more years to your life and life to your years and simultaneously allow you to grow into your excellence. The importance of getting your heart pumping with some physical exercise cannot be overlooked!

Benefits of Physical Exercise

Our bodies love to move! We are designed to move. It is not a coincidence that when we exercise, our bodies release endorphins (the "feel good chemicals"), which help reduce stress and boost our mood. Our bodies will reward us for exercising. As indicated above, exercise (moving) causes our body to release the feel-good hormone endorphins, which improves our mood and, by extension, the interpretation of events and challenges we face. To encourage the release of endorphins, we need to start moving.

In our modern lives, we tend to live a more sedentary life, which differs from our previous outdoor style of living when we had to hunt for our food. Technology is making it easier to work and communicate.

43

However, with these advances have also come a more sedentary lifestyle. We are spending an unprecedented amount of time in front of screens, either working or entertaining ourselves. Being inactive for extended periods of time has resulted in lifestyle-related diseases such as obesity, diabetes, and high blood pressure. More people simply drive from point A to point B, although there has been a recent drive for more exercise or physical activity. There is a move to make communities more bike-friendly by the creation of bike paths and by increasing access routes or paths for pedestrians. These moves are commendable since by improving the safety of pedestrians and cyclists, society is encouraging a more active, outdoor style of living. All the reasons mentioned above should be commended because it is a step in the right direction to improving your health and simultaneously adding years to your life and life to your years while you grow into your excellence.

Physical activity also sets you up for success by encouraging restful sleep and if you are looking to lose weight. Maintaining a healthy weight is part of your revival. Sometimes, the missing piece of the puzzle for individuals on a weight loss journey could be sufficient exercise. It is simply not enough to change your diet. When physical activity becomes part of your lifestyle, your efforts, and any weight loss you experience are maintained over the months and years. Your metabolism changes as you age, and being physically active helps boost your metabolism and, therefore, maintain your weight well into your golden years. As one ages, other health challenges emerge, and these may encourage a more sedentary life. Let us explore what exercises we can employ if we are experiencing painful knees.

With painful knees, walking, running, jumping, and squatting, though all exercises may aggravate knee joint pains. Better exercise choices for clients experiencing knee joint pains would be cycling and swimming. Swimming exercises the whole body whilst supporting the body because of the buoyancy of the water. This will remove any stress on your knees, though the movement of your body parts will occur, giving you all the benefits of walking or running.

Physical exercise is not only necessary for your health but also vital. It is a practice necessary to add years to your life and life to years. It improves your mood and generally causes you to be more pleasant to be around. Exercise not only improves your physical health, but also your mental health and spirit all benefit from exercise. Let us examine the main types of physical exercise and their benefits. If you don't already have an exercise regime, I want to offer you a strong starting point. If exercise is already part of your life, you may find yourself always enjoying cardio-based exercise as opposed to resistance training. I want to give you some insight into the importance of keeping both aerobics and strength training in balance.

Types of Exercise and the Importance of Intensity

Since we are focusing on ensuring you add years to your life and life to your years, I'd suggest we examine basic aerobic and strength training exercises. Both categories can be broken down further into many subgenres, but let's start with an overview so that you may feel inspired. I am especially looking to those of you who may not have a regular exercise routine. A weekly exercise routine is necessary for reviving your body, it is attainable, and it can be fun!

When looking at your weekly aerobic needs, you may already be contributing to them without even realizing it. About 150 minutes of *brisk* walking, swimming, biking, gardening, or even weekly lawn mowing is all it takes to start a routine. Alternatively, if your fitness level is already at a proficient level, you may want to engage in activities that are more rigorous and challenging (after consulting with your doctor to ensure you are approaching a new routine safely). This can look like aerobic dancing or running for 75 min/week. If you have the time and motivation, or if you feel you would like a further challenge, incorporating three hundred minutes (5 hours) per week will really be effective. Do not do yourself a disservice by negating this amount of aerobic exercise. You can easily do 5 hours a week by doing a bit every day and starting new daily healthy exercise habits. Over the course of a week, you will see that your efforts can really add up!

Now, let us not forget about strength training. Strengthening all your major muscle groups with weight training will require repetitions a minimum of two times per week. You can use free weights or weight machines, but if those are not available to you, simply engage in activities where your own weight resistance is utilized, such as using a pull-up bar or rock climbing. Heavy gardening may even be appropriate here. Just remember it can be as simple as using your own weight as resistance, whatever that may look like. (If you need suggestions there are a plethora of resources online.)

The effectiveness of both aerobic exercise and strength training comes down to your intensity level when moving. There is quite a difference between going for a leisurely walk and going for a brisk walk when it comes to affecting your health. For maximum benefit, your activity level should be at a moderate or vigorous level of intensity. However, what this feels like is based solely on the individual, as everyone is at a different level of physical fitness. What may be a challenging routine for one person may feel easy to the next. A safe way to begin gauging this is by assessing your breathing while working out. When you moderately exert yourself, you will break a sweat after about 12 minutes and will feel comfortable having a conversation but have difficulty singing. When participating in more vigorous activity, you will break a sweat after five to seven minutes of your workout, and you will only be able to express yourself in short sentences or words, needing to stop and catch your breath more often.

Using these guidelines is a fantastic way to really assess where you are at with your exertion levels. You may also monitor your heart rate, of course, but you will require a heart monitoring system attached to you (ex., a Fitbit or something similar) or must stop to do calculations on the spot. I like to keep things straightforward and simply just connect with my breathing.

Please keep in mind that you can always *over*exert yourself. If you find that you are short of breath or are experiencing chest pains, it is usually an indication of working beyond your capacity. There is a fine line between engaging in vigorous activity and pushing yourself too far. Know where your physical threshold is and build up your stamina and strength step by step over time. This is a lifelong practice, so I urge you to be mindful and stay safe. As you can see, you do not need a lot, if any, equipment to start an exercise program. All you need is to get out of your own way!

Reflection:

Do I have a physical fitness routine?

What do I tend to lean towards, aerobic activity or strength training?

How can I incorporate more physical fitness activity into my day and week?

How can I make being more physically active a priority?

_____

_____

_____

_____

_____

_____

_____

_____

_____

_____

The Importance of Rest

Rest is essential to our physical well-being and all levels of our revival if you are to grow into your excellence. Many interpret rest as being intrusive to their daily plans. Some may even try to judge the recipient of rest as being lazy or trying to avoid work. On the contrary, you require rest to work at your highest potential (be it physically or otherwise). Rest allows for recovery, resuscitation, repair, rebuild, and restoration of the physical body and mind. Resting improves cardiovascular health, lowers blood pressure, and reduces levels of the stress hormone cortisol. Your mood, alertness, mental clarity, creativity, and motivation are all improved with rest (which in turn improves your productivity and quality of your life). Vacations specifically reduce the risk of heart disease and increase your lifespan.

We work long hours to keep on top of our growing workloads, running the risk of stress and burnout in the process, as we desperately try to keep up. Vacations become a second thought as we battle stress, illness, and the constant pressure to find time for all our commitments outside work. Rest is an essential part of doing our best work and being more productive at work. According to the Institute for Work and Families, fewer than half of U.S. employees take all their vacation days, and Glassdoor reported that 61% of employees work during vacation. Individuals tend to think of vacation as an indulgence that we cannot afford, but it is a necessary part of doing your best work.

Various authors have indicated the benefits of taking a vacation and have advanced at least eight benefits of taking a vacation:

1. The office is not a place for inspiration, so getting away gives you an opportunity to draw on your creativity.

2. Leaving the office moves you away from your comfort zone, thereby giving you an opportunity for a different perspective.

3. Your health benefits enormously. One study showed that 82% of small business owners who took a vacation were performing better at work when they returned. As a bonus, about a third of men who took a vacation were less likely to die of heart disease.

4. It allows your brain to get a break from this continued daily grind that the office environment presents.

5. You may not realize it, but a change of scenery is necessary as it strangely gives new life to your endeavors.

6. It facilitates networking.

7. It allows you to realize that the office can function without you, thereby facilitating the delegation and minimizes of the stress that comes with overworking yourself.

8. It keeps both yourself and your workers happy. It allows them to recognize their importance to the company and will encourage them to do their best work.

Sleep is one of the most important aspects of rest as it allows you to regenerate not only your physical self but your mind and spirit as well. Experts tell us that there are two basic types of sleep. Rapid eye movement sleep and non-rapid eye movement sleep. The non-rapid eye movement sleep has three stages. Stage 1 is the changeover from wakefulness to sleep; stage 2 is the period of light sleep before entering stage 3, which is deep sleep. It is during deep sleep that glucose metabolism in the brain increases, supporting both short- and long-term memory and overall learning. It is during deep sleep that the pituitary gland in the brain secretes growth hormones, which leads to growth and development of the body. Deep sleep allows for other benefits such as energy restoration, cell regeneration, and the blood supply to muscles is increased, tissues, and bones are repaired, and the immune system is strengthened.

Sleep

We must distinguish between rest or relaxation and sleep. In our daily experience, we note that our productivity declines on the day following a night without restful sleep. We spend that day abusing coffee and energy drinks, but our productivity is still sub-optimal. In the elderly who get by on fewer hours of sleep, we observe them stumble through the following day and are quick to attribute their stumbles to growing old, but is there more to it?

The result of no sleep or insufficient sleep causes one to stumble along the following day. There are more ominous repercussions to a deficiency in sleep. There is an increase in inflammatory markers and the stress hormone cortisol. Cerebrospinal fluid functions in cleaning the brain. During sleep, the channels within the brain dilate physiologically and allow for a more intimate association between brain cells and the cleansing cerebrospinal fluid. In experiments with mice, when asleep, the cerebrospinal fluid was exchanged twenty-fold. Researchers measured a

60% increase in the flow of cerebrospinal fluid when mice were asleep compared to when they were awake. Recognizing that 20% of the energy used by our body is by the brain, the brain performs quite an arduous task, during which it generates a lot of waste. Therefore, cleaning is vital if the brain is to do its best work.

People who are sleep-deprived have increased levels of inflammatory markers in circulation. If unchecked, the inflammation will have serious health consequences and contribute to heart disease, cancer, and brain diseases, such as Alzheimer's disease.

We recommend that adults get six to eight hours of sleep each night, no excuses! You must be mindful and obtain an uninterrupted, restful sleep each night to constantly feel alert and refreshed. Therefore, it is ideal that you create a solid sleep regime for yourself. This starts by committing to start winding down a minimum of 45 min before you would like to sleep. Start this time by avoiding any distractions (for example, pets, TV, discussions with partners, anything to do with your phone, etc.) and allowing your mind to begin a process of relaxation. A warm shower or bath can help you to begin to relax for bedtime. A cup of warm almond milk, as well as ensuring your bedroom is an appropriate temperature for sleep (no cooler than 20°C or 68°F). Be mindful that the absence of light (or very dim light) will trigger the production of the hormone melatonin, which is essential for your sleep/wake cycle. Calm and gentle music, as well as pink noise, can help you relax and drift off to sleep (personal taste can vary with this, and I suggest you investigate as there are many free online resources). Getting serious about cultivating and sticking to your sleep regime will be a game changer in your life. Remember, the objective is to facilitate your growth into your excellence.

Beyond sleep, it is also ideal to have one full day of rest a week. This allows you to slow down with the benefit of self-revival. When you rest by taking a day off from your usual schedule, you will gain increased drive and inspiration for the tasks that lie ahead. This is built into your regular calendars with the weekend days. It is rare to work all seven days of the week and taking at least one day over the weekend for rest and play is ideal. A day off for rest does not simply imply that you laze about or sleep for that day. Resting can look like changing your focus on that day and engaging in something other than work, be it playing a game, relaxing with friends, or spending quality time with family. It is a rest from your daily chores and, therefore, will serve to re-energize you and provide you with useful mental relaxation.

Cultivating a strong relationship with both exercise and rest is essential. Creating this balance will allow you to sustain a definitive tempo in your days, as opposed to a cycle of burnout and then the need to recover. Your energy is sustained daily, and your life will improve dramatically.

Reflection:

How much sleep do I get on average?

Do I have healthy sleep habits?

How do I feel about taking a break or an actual day off to rest and enjoy myself?

How easy is it to drift off to sleep?

What distractions interfere with my ability to drift off to sleep?

How can I improve the quality of my restful sleep?

How do I make downtime in my life?

_____

_____

_____

_____

_____

_____

_____

_____

_____

Temperance

Everyone deserves to enjoy life to the fullest! "Eat, drink, and be merry!" is advised. Reflect on the last time you overindulged. Was it eating too much of your favorite food? Or having too much to drink? How did it make you feel? When you throw yourself into anything with total abandon, it is more difficult to exercise self-control, and having discipline, thus preventing overindulgence, is essential to facilitate your growth into your excellence. Exercising temperance is necessary to add years to your life and life to your years. Avoiding excess in all areas of your life is essential for healthy living. Practicing self-control is like anything: the more you practice it, the better you become at it.

What is temperance? This is the quality of moderation or self-restraint. Human beings lack the practice of temperance in their lives, either because of ignorance or from a lack of self-control. Interestingly, the feeling of temperance is found within. Your body will send you strong signals when you are at the line of "enough." It is up to you to learn how to hear and feel these signals. For example, you are eating your favorite meal, You may finish half your plate and feel quite satisfied, but you keep eating anyway because it tastes so good. After clearing your dish by eating all that was placed on it, instead of feeling just full and satisfied, you feel overly full and uncomfortable. You are now wishing you had stopped when you felt satisfied. Your body knows its limits, and it expects you to listen!

The practice of temperance easily extends into all aspects of one's life. We previously talked about physical activity. This is an area where temperance becomes important as well. If you overexert yourself and you push beyond your own limits, this may cause injury. If you over-exercise and do not give your muscles enough time to recover and repair, the risk of injury increases. Temperance is an essential practice in the achievement of your goals. Exercise regimes include both aerobic and strength training; swinging back and forth between the two in equal measure demonstrates balance.

The catholic catechism describes temperance as the moral virtue that moderates the attraction of pleasure and provides balance. Again, it is not about denying yourself pleasure but about developing mastery of your own will. Anything done in excess invariably has an adverse effect on our bodies. It is your responsibility to take temperance into consideration when engaging in any activity. It is a fine balance to find within, but I assure you when you find this balance. You will feel fantastic and reap all the benefits that temperance has to offer. Your body will reward you with a vibrancy like you have never experienced before, and you will continue to feel good throughout the years as you grow into your excellence!

Reflection

In what areas in your life does balance come easy?

Where do you feel you push too hard and overextend yourself?

Where do you feel you push too little and not meet your own potential?

How can you apply more temperance in your life starting today?

What does temperance look like in your life on a grander scale?

_____

_____

_____

_____

_____

_____

_____

_____

_____

We have finished examining the various aspects of reviving our physical bodies, a prerequisite to allow your growth into your excellence. We discussed the importance of choosing the right foods to fuel your body and how that may contribute to your world beyond your plate. We touched upon our relationship with sunlight and fresh air. The importance of moving your body was highlighted, we explored the value of rest to our body, and we addressed the value of temperance to our body and how it's all about creating balance in your life and fostering your growth into your excellence.

I hope you are feeling inspired to cultivate changes in your relationship to your physical self so that you may live your daily life with vitality and joy as you grow into your excellence. Remember, your body works *with* you, not against you. We need to develop a strong relationship with our body and its needs. Appropriate self-care ensures your body will serve you for years to come as you grow into excellence!

In part two of this book, we will move on to exploring the next component of the triune: your mind. We will explore and uncover the relationship you have with your mind so that you may nourish it appropriately to cultivate its revival and facilitate your growth into your excellence. Of course, this will start with discussing what the mind is! It is not something you can see or feel, but it is an integral part of you, nonetheless. Working on the revival of your mind is the next step to adding years to your life and life to your years as you grow into your excellence.

PART TWO: THE MIND

Have you ever wondered about the impact of your mind on your behavior, character, and your body? In medical school doctors recall the attempts by professors to consider some illnesses as psychosomatic illness. Simply put this describes the impact of the mind in causing the body to experience ill health. The impact of the mind on our beings is probably best memorialized by the negro poet Cowper, in his 1788 poem, the Negro's Complaint, in his reflection on the dehumanizing effects of slavery, this Caucasian gentleman was able to keep his chin up in his poem an extract of which went as follows…. *'Still in thoughts as free as ever, what are England's rights I ask, me from my delights to sever, me to torture, me to task? Fleecy locks and black complexion cannot forfeit nature's claim; skins may differ, but affection dwells in whites and blacks the same. If I were so tall as to reach the pole or to grasp the ocean at a span, I must be measured by my soul, the mind is the standard of the man.'* Dr Martin Luther King endorsed the role of the mind through his use of bits of Negro poet Cowper writings in his speeches. Other authors and professors have addressed the same concept in different ways, for example Professor Roy Meadow postulated the term Munchausen Syndrome by proxy which by extension massages the concept of the power of the mind over the body. It is therefore not farfetched to explore the role of the working of the mind in the evolution of the healthiest and best version of oneself. Muhammad Ali understood the importance of the workings of the mind as embodied in his reflective statement…..*"I hated every minute of training, but I said, don't quit. Suffer now and live the rest of your life as a champion." – Muhammad Ali*

59

We at Philburn Academy will help you to understand this concept and seek to massage your mindset to allow you to evolve into the healthiest version of you, as we the proponents of the BMS ecosystem realize the critical role played by the mind in the success of this approach. A simple belief about yourself permeates every aspect of your life.

Again and again, we see the attempt by our fellow men to dull the impact of their minds by exposing themselves to a plethora of mind altering substances, be it alcohol or other harmful drugs, marijuana, cocaine and its various cousins in an attempt to undergo a mental drift away from the effects of a functioning mind, some people may claim this mental drift as an attempt to step away from reality. Surely there is a personality type that is drawn to that type of behavior, yet the substances used, though they eventually affect the body, the primary purpose is for immediacy of the mind alteration that results from the use of these substances.

Would you therefore, as a minimum, appreciate the evidence. That our minds play a governing role over our bodies? Its appropriate guidance will be immeasurable in our journeys of becoming the healthiest, most active versions of ourselves. In a nutshell, therefore, our foods consumed take care of or is supposed to take care of our physical bodies, but our mind governs our thought process, and the combination creates the image that society chooses to refer to as our personality.

It is based on the impact of this thought process that people differ. We will describe our sporting champion in one light, our successful businessmen in a different light, successful relationships may also be viewed in a different light, and we are even sold tools to allow us to reap successes in certain endeavors, but on closer analysis though the recipe may differ the acquisition of the desired outcome lies in the sandwich of mindset.

Why is it that you feel fear when breaking new ground, or in common parlance getting out of your comfort zone? Yet there are many people moving forward anyways despite this fear? Einstein is credited with the truism that nothing happens until something moves. Yet many, including myself, would introduce a slight alteration to Einstein view to read nothing happens until the mind evolves, usually through the acquisition of new experiences in the school of life. In this section I want to explore the second component of the BMS ecosystem. The second step is all about your mind and how you can create changes to continue building yourself in line with adding years to your life and life to your years as you grow into your excellence. Let us first discuss exactly what the mind is in an individual.

Chapter 6: An Introduction to Your Mind

*"**The sky is not the limit. Your mind is.**"*Marilyn Munroe

The trained mind is a rich mind. Robert Kiyosaki

The Mind

Inherent in Kiyosaki's statement, the mind can be trained. Even before our time mankind grappled with trying to find a reason why people differ. Through the ages, various hypotheses have been advanced, among them phrenology a field of study which looks at the conformation of the skull as an indication of mental faculties and character traits, others focus on craniology, here the size and shape of the head is used as a sort of predictor of mental faculties and character traits. The discussion continues and now has evolved into, is it nature (genes) or is it the environment (nurture) that determines who we become? Irrespective of your allegiance, I prefer to think that both contribute and likely in variable amounts. Thus, the final product cannot be fully attributed to nature, nor can it be purely because of the environment. It is the contribution of the environment that Kiyosaki seems to be talking about. I believe Gilbert Gottlieb, the eminent neuroscientist puts it best, he says, 'not only do genes and environment cooperate as we develop, but the genes require input from the environment to work well.

It is now emerging that people have capacity for lifelong learning and brain development, if that is so, then since our genetic endowment is fixed; we have the potential for growth with time because of the impact of the environment. The interaction between the fixed genetic endowment and the capacity and willingness for change. Effective learning makes change inevitable, so mankind continues to metamorphosize with time. It is on this basis we believe that the BMS ecosystem can add years to your life and life to your years because of its teachings. Once you understand and implement the concepts, we expect the results to be a longer and more active life. If I may burrow the words of Robert Sternberg, one perceived to be an intelligence expert, he postulates that the major factor in whether people achieve excellence is not some fixed prior ability, but purposeful engagement. Binet recognized that those who start out the smartest may not end up the smartest. Indicating strongly that training/ the environment can effect change in outcome. The mind is therefore not a fixed construct.

What is the actual mind? Where does it live and how does it serve us? What is its relationship to the other components of self (the body and spirit)? Some have described the mind as the set of cognitive faculties including consciousness, imagination, perception, thinking, judgement, language, and memory, which is housed in the brain. It allows for imagination, recognition and appreciation and contributes to feelings and emotions. So again, the brain is the physical mass that is a part of our body systems and houses the mind. Yet the mind exists within its own realm and is intertwined with the physical being as well as the spirit.

How is it that while one person may be willing to step forward and continue to grow as a person, even in the face of fear, another may shrink? What exactly is this unique differentiating character with which some seem to be gifted? We all feel fear when trying something new. It is part of our human experience! There are two types of people. Ones that tend to always be looking back, blaming others, or constantly looking at the negative side of things and the others who think positively. Positive thinking as Zig Ziglar contends will let you do everything better than negative thinking will. Albert Einstein advises that we stay away from negative people because they have a problem for every solution. Those who say the glass is half full are the positive thinkers and are willing to take a risk and believe that there are always better opportunities for themselves. With some commitment, desire, and application, they strive to move the glass from being half full to full or fuller. What is the driving force in these people? It is their minds, and more specifically their **mindset**. The view one adapts to their life affects the way they live their life. It can determine whether you become the person you want to be and what you accomplish.

If you believe your qualities are fixed, then you are burdened by the need to prove yourself. For example, if one continues to tell a child that he or she is smart, then it does something to the child's mind making it difficult to address challenges or failures. Similarly, by telling a child that he is foolish, it will cause the child to accept failure and suboptimal performances as his best result since his condition essentially places a sealing on just how much he/she is able to achieve. Considering the room for growth afforded by nurture, are we then mere unprocessed material which should be shaped by nurture? Should we accept that we at any stage of our lives are mere foundations on which much can be built? We are of the view that growth is possible in all, but it requires desire and application. It is therefore impossible to predict or know a person's true potential, it is impossible to know what can be accomplished with years of passion, toil, and training. If you have the passion for having years added to your life and life to your years and you are willing to work at it, with the appropriate training you will get there and so grow into your excellence. The history of mankind is replete with countless stories of folks who were considered just average by their peers and even advised to seek a career in other disciplines with application, hard work and training they exceeded many an expectation. Of recent memory is Michael Jordan, the American basketball player, who did not make his high school basketball team, this he claims ignited a passion within him and now years later he is revered around the world as the greatest basketball player of all times.

Examination of your mindset is not a modern concept. Throughout the ages the inquiry of mindset has been a constant in human study. Time and time again there have been writings and reflections on the adverse reactions of people who blame other people or things for not moving forward or why they may not have had more of an opportunity extended to them. One such story that really highlights this for me is the Parable of Talents that we find in the Bible. This is a great example of someone squandering a great opportunity, with the classic behavior of a negative thinker, finding excuses, solely because of their mindset.

The Parable of Talents

In the Parable of Talents, the story is told of a rich man who had three servants. Upon departure for a trip, he gave each of his servants a portion of his riches in talents. (Talents here refer to money in the form of seed capital thought to each be worth a modern sum of over a million dollars!) The first servant is given five talents, the second given three talents and the third servant given one. The master tells them to care for his money and the first two servants go forth and use their talents to trade and gain profit. When the master returns, they can give him back double the talents with which they were entrusted! He is so impressed that he gives them back some of the money, which for his servants is a life changing gift no doubt. However, the third servant, fearful of the gift, simply hides/ buries the talent and returns it as is to the master upon his return. The master scolds and chides him for not being willing to take advantage of investing and trying to create profit, even with only one talent.

There was no observable difference between the servants themselves. The only difference was their mindset and how they viewed the gifts given to them. The first two servants saw their glasses as half *full*, **an opportunity,** and went forward with enthusiasm and curiosity to try to fill the glass. The third, however, wasted an opportunity to invest and grow, because to him, the glass was half empty. He then had to do everything that he could to prevent the glass from becoming empty, to him his safest option was to bury the talent with which he was entrusted. May I ask you are you burying your talents? There was no self-motivation. Was it because of his mindset that he was left with nothing? Take some time to begin observing people around you. Study people at your work, places of worship, even people in the public space. You will begin to clearly see a distinction between two types of mindsets. In simplest terms, some will see the glass half full, an opportunity to fill the glass and the others will see the glass as half empty fearful that they may lose the contents of the glass and render it empty; creating difficulty with a granted opportunity.

Let us look at the scenario a bit more closely. Firstly, we are not all given equal opportunities. A single opportunity should be sufficient. We are alive which is one opportunity, that is all we need, **LIFE is the opportunity we need,** to grow into our greatness. The same object being looked at by two different individuals came up with different perspectives. The major difference seems to be their mindset and the interpretation of what they see. It is particularly intuitive that one individual sees the glass with a positive outlook, the glass is half full, inherently, suggesting the possibility of filling it up. The other perspective was the glass being half empty, empty here being a negative connotation and by extension an indication of the mindset. The interpretations suggest one of hope and opportunity whilst the other suggest one of fear and the need for protection. The one of hope and opportunity sees the half full glass with the hope that it can be filled if the right steps are taken. The other who sees the glass as half empty seems to be paralyzed with fear that the glass is almost empty, it is halfway there so any action that he undertakes may result in the glass becoming empty. Hence the need to protect it. Hide it or even bury it, if you will, as in the story of the talents above. Our mindsets therefore go a long way in determining how we interpret what we see and guide our next steps.

Reflection:

Why would a glass being half full motivate?

Why would a glass being half empty discourage?

Are you willing to work with the gifts that you are given?

Who in your life sees the glass half full?

Who sees it half empty?

How are you affected by their behavior?

Have you ever blamed someone or something else for something in your life instead of taking ownership or responsibility for it?

_____

_____

_____

_____

_____

_____

_____

_____

The Influences of The Mind

As we mentioned, the brain is the physical mass that is a part of our body system and houses the mind. The mind exists within its own realm, and greatly affects our physical being. This is why it is imperative to understand your mind and how it works so that you may work on its revival, as you did with the body. (Never forget that everything is interconnected!)

The body is a mere vehicle for the carriage of our minds and spirit, so our bodies are mere vessels which are directed by our minds and to some degree our spirit guides the direction of the mind which gives rise to our personality, beliefs, and traits. Recall that the negro poet Cowper long told us the mind is the standard of the man.

To connect with your mind, you must first fully understand that the truths which you perceive around you first begin with your mind and it is colored by the world around you that is constantly relaying negativity towards you and it is your mind, conditioned by your spirit, that will decide what we do with this negativity. This starts right from the time you were born with the closest people around you while growing up (your family, teachers, and caretakers) and continues into your adulthood. Obviously, our family and caretakers thought they were doing an outstanding job of protecting us from ourselves, a role now employed by an aspect of the mind called the ego. Arguably, the ego is something that has been formed from your conditioning and habits. This is the protective or rational part of the mind. It basically restrains us or seeks to restrain us from risky behavior. Based on the workings of the ego, it seems that we live in a society that is flooded with negativity. We are constantly being sent messages on what we can and cannot do, and what we must do to be happy, the message in a nutshell advises us to remain in our comfort zones. A clear message from the ego. At times these messages can really be seen as some sort of negative plot against your dreams and desires! I am sure that you have met people in your life who simply claim certain career paths or activities are "just not for them". I am sure that if you had the opportunity to hear the origin of that belief, you would hear stories about childhood, school, family life and even about one's peers that were fraught with discouragement as opposed to supporting the individual with their dreams or ideas. (Perhaps you may even relate to this!) This person continues to grow up into a society where following your dreams is not encouraged and the focus becomes all about staying in your lane and remaining comfortable. All in all, there is a focus on negativity as opposed to positivity. It all feels like some sort of evil plot by society against ensuring people are truly happy and sharing positivity. This negativity versus positivity is boxed in two separate mind sets, a fixed or negative mindset versus a growth or positive mindset.

Interpretation of thoughts or saying is colored by the mindset enshrouded by the spirit. As seen above in the parable, two servants interpreted their gift as an opportunity for growth, but one saw it as an opportunity to protect.

Seeing the ego is such a dominant force in carving our personality, is there any guidance to be had to help us overcome the control of the ego?

Overcoming the Ego

You are the only one capable of overcoming the limitations of your ego, to do so some self-insight is important. You may need to recalibrate your thought process which may result in you becoming less offended by criticism. The more attention placed on criticism, the more defensive you become which can lead to you becoming quarrelsome, with the resultant toll that has on your energy and focus.

There is no need to go through life with the persistent need to win or to be right, this may muddy the contact with your true self. Since self-reflection in this circumstance may be a blur.

Deepak Chopra advises that we must go beyond the constant clamor of ego, beyond the tools of logic and reason, to the still, calm place within us: The realm of the soul.

Though the ego is protective, it also enjoys judging and comparing others to you. We should strive to vacate the seat of superiority or inferiority. This serves no useful purpose apart from resenting others, it encourages confrontation and hostility among people. This rubs you from life's true enjoyment.

Overcoming the ego leads to a type of internal peace which is based on satisfaction. The craving for accomplishments and more can be silenced by overcoming the ego.

Since the protection extended to us by the ego tries to keep us in our comfort zone and tries to ensure that we are safe, would there be any need to override it? Sticking to the persistence of the ego, we will not venture outside our comfort zones and will seek to keep our being from risk taking and challenges, but unless we challenge ourselves, we do not grow, the fixed mindset is simply an enemy of personal growth.

People will be inspired to act in accordance with their beliefs (be it negative or positive). This is how your **mindset** is generated. Boiled down to its simplest platform, your mindset governs the way in which you handle a situation. There are two mindsets we can possess: a **fixed mindset** or negative mindset and a **growth mindset or positive**. As with our bodies, our minds also require nourishment and an optimal environment in which to flourish. There of course will also be factors which impact our mind. We will discuss these in turn as well as distinguish between both the fixed and growth mindsets so that you may understand which you possess and what is optimal for living a life filled with more vitality and thus help you to grow into your excellence.

Reflection:

What are some negative messages you receive daily?

Can you identify any aspect in your life which has been influenced by naysayers?

Now that you understand how the people around you influence you, how do you plan to address this situation?

Which do you consider is most useful in your life comfort or creativity?

_____

_____

_____

_____

_____

_____

_____

_____

Let us begin with the importance of nourishing our mind for the better. We will further examine the growth and fixed mindset and come to fully understand how your life can be affected by each mindset. I will offer you some clear reflection and guidance on taking care of your mind.

Chapter 7: Boxed In

Becoming is better than being. The fixed mindset does not allow people the luxury of becoming. You already have to be. — Carol Dweck

Entrapment

We are groomed by society to fit into a particular box. What do I mean? I hear you ask.

Whether we recognize it or not from birth, society has placed us into some group with expectations on how we are supposed to behave. We have seen the continued rebellion by babies and toddlers to confinement. Yet society continues along with its conscious or unconscious desire to box us in. This, it usually does by attaching labels to us, we are told for example that we are smart, or we are foolish, there is no hope for us etc. These statements in essence help to shape our mindsets by inducing a belief system in us that helps to shape our attitude to several different life experiences. Our attitude emanates from a belief system which cultivates a type of behavior that evolves into a habit from which a personality type is developed. In this scenario results are amplified or explained. One may argue that through the application of labels, society has some expectations of us. Unfortunately for those applying labels, a person's true potential is unknown and cannot be known, because it is unlikely for someone else to be able to predict what you can become with years of passion, hard work, support, and guidance.

Yet we see this practice flourish in society. We have an unconscious but active desire to place people into groups. Parents, for example, will place their children in a group either inadvertently or willingly. From the simple refence of our children as being smart, the comparison begins, I am smart, because of what my parents told me. Does that therefore mean that I am smarter and thus superior to little Johnnie? If we hold on to this thought, with time it becomes our belief and so we develop the habit (belief held for a long time) which will merge into a personality type and a mindset. So, by the simple, maybe idle chatter to the little ones about how smart they are can have some pervasive consequences in how he/she feels about himself and how he/she responds to challenges. It may also define the amount of effort expended to complete a task. It may be seen that because he is smart, he does not have to try and when or if he does poorly, he either tries to explain his short comings by blaming something or someone but never himself, alternatively he may tell himself that because 'he has it', he does not have to try. For clarity let us view the impact of this language on two individuals and the impact it may have on them. (a) Say Melissa is continuously showered with sweet nothingness about how smart she is, that may eventually lull her into believing that she must accept the label and behave in the manner expected from the label that has been applied to her. She must act in a manner to give credence to the label. She has been boxed in! Mindset creation, the development of a fixed mindset. As a result, any time she is faced with a challenge or potential failure, since that goes against her belief system, (She is smart, she does not have to try) she tries to avoid the challenge, she needs to reassure herself that she is smart. Failure is not an option. Melissa needs to preserve the hand that she believes that she has been dealt, that hand 'smartness', must be validated by her actions and behavior. So, your entire being is about self-revalidation, consciously or unconsciously you go forth embarking on this journey in which you subscribe to the label placed on you, you try to protect that label. On the other hand, unlike Melissa, if Johnnie has done something well instead of telling him how smart he is and that he is obviously talented. Show recognition for his effort. Something like well-done Johnnie, I like your effort in completing the task, I am impressed. The difference being Melissa will leave with the view that she is smart, (her talent being smartness) whereas the message to Johnnie in a nutshell is clear, you are able to achieve with effort. This will help Johnnie accept that to achieve there must be effort. So, though he has the raw material needed to succeed, effort is required. I refer you back to parable above of the talents/gifts received by the servants. In the case of the servant who received the one talent, his immediate desire was to protect it and in so doing he buried it. By labelling individuals what are we burying?

The Phenomenon of Tiptoeing

If we accept that by labelling individuals, we are burying somethings, we will understand that to move out from this burial box, we need to break through, this thought has been expressed in numerous ways by many, we hear talk about breaking through the proverbial glass ceiling etc. which may be another way of referring to breaking through the box, a phenomenon much like tiptoeing. You see with tiptoeing you need a base, much like the balls of your feet but with your heels raised; the effect is a small gain in height, sufficient to crash that proverbial glass ceiling. Looked at another way, having that base you have a starting point from which you, through tiptoeing can grow. So by approaching the little ones with effort centric praise as opposed to an innate factor that you may suggest they possess, such as talent which is equivalent to labels, we may see a drift away from being boxed in and we may come to understand that the gifts or talents that we have been dealt is a mere template from which to grow, hence the creation of a different mindset, not that you are endowed with unchangeable characteristics but rather you have the necessary raw materials which through the exercise of passion, hard work, support, and guidance you can morph into anything your heart desires, thus demonstrating the growth mindset and allowing you to grow into your excellence. No one has accurate self-insight into their assets and limitations. Though I posit that one can grow using the raw materials with which he/she is endowed, it is obvious that in the process of growth you need guidance, support, training, belief, and commitment that it can be done. With this belief system you will be able to convert life setbacks into future successes.

It stands to reason that with the culture of applying labels, not only are we boxing in individuals we are also burying opportunities. I believe that my former student Doctor Pastor Miles Munroe was right when he spoke of the cemetery as being the wealthiest place on earth. Why, do I hear you ask? It is simply because buried within the box, the walls of the cemetery are dreams unfulfilled, opportunities not explored, books not written, and talents not developed. The mind is therefore a potent component of your being and a necessary component of the Triune. Even though it is carried around on the body, it directs the body's activities, so it is important that we are honest with it and nourish it appropriately, if we are to grow into our excellence.

The Power of Praise

To praise an individual is inevitable, not only can it encourage, but it also ensures recognition for the task for which you are praised. Many superficially would ask; why not, we all need to feel that we are encouraged and acknowledged for what we do. Looking at it in this manner may cause a penetrating discomfort based on the manner and what is praised. If your praise is result based, the evidence is that this type of praise boxes you in, analogous to attachment of labels, the result a fixed mindset, In Johnnie's case, the praise is effort based and he comes to appreciate the value of effort and so admires a challenge, the creation of a different mindset, the growth mindset. A necessary disposition to facilitate you growing into your excellence.

We are therefore saying that praise does not box you in, what boxes you in is being praised; are you praising result and silently tying it to talent or are you praising the approach and appreciating the effort involved in to get there?

The danger of praising results and making it seem that you are a natural, that you seem to have a certain gift or talent has the ill effect of stereotyping you and therefore boxes you in with a certain type of mindset that expects a certain type of behavior from you. This is not only limiting but it causes you not to expend effort to allow you to grow into your excellence. Your effort is spent trying to live according to your understanding of what that label or stereotype expects from you. You are trying to live the life someone has carved out for you. In trying to live someone's expectation of you, you fail to live your reality and in so doing your behavior is controlled by that stereotype/label. Your actions, including lying, are designed to maintain that stereotype. If the stereotype is positive your activity is designed to try to maintain it, if it is a negative label, you become fearful of deserving it.

This labelling therefore keeps you in a state of anxiety fearful that the results of your activity may either cause you to lose your place in that stereotyped position, if the stereotype can be seen as positive or if the results of your activity don't quite lead to results that is expected in that stereotyped space, it may lead to a sense of worthlessness and a sense of not belonging to that label.

Stereotyping is viewed as the offspring of prejudice. This though is only based on someone's view of you and must not be lived out by you. The approach to this prejudice by the growth mindset is different. It is confronted with confidence, you see it as a challenge which your abilities will allow you to surmount.

Reflections:

Do you feel boxed in?

Does society have unfair expectations of your abilities?

Do you feel that despite your best efforts you are unable to shake society's expectations of you?

Do you believe that Talent outshines effort?

Do you believe one is only able to achieve based on his/her talents?

Is praise good or bad?

How should we praise our children?

_____

_____

_____

_____

_____

_____

_____

_____

_____

Chapter 8: The Tentacles of our Creation

What allowed me to take the first step to choose growth and risk rejection? In the fixed mindset, I needed my blame and bitterness. It made me feel more righteous, powerful, and whole than thinking that I was at fault. The growth mindset allowed me to give up the blame and move on. The growth mindset gave me a mother. — Carol S. Dweck

The Dynamic

As is evident from the discussion above, we are a product of the interplay between our genetics, colloquially referred to as our DNA and our environment. An interaction between Nature and Nurture. Obviously as we grow older, arguably our environment should have a greater role in who we become, but we know or expect a seed to give rise to the plant from which it arose. So, though the plant is the product of the seed, the seed is the important predecessor of the plant, but not only that the seed is dependent on its immediate environment to blossom and grow into a plant. Similarly, our mindset is developed because of the interplay between our pluripotential raw material with which we are born and how it is massaged.

As family, teachers, coaches, and support personnel, we may be guilty of massaging the little ones with pleasantries which unknowingly leads to the creation of the mindset which when fully developed extends its tentacles to all aspects of their lives. This phenomenon, an integral and necessary component of the triune directs and guides who we become. Through the extension of its tentacles, it influences every aspect of our person rightly or wrongly. It determines how we interpret what we are exposed to, it determines how we interact with people in the workspace, it determines how we respond to life challenges and irrespective of how we present ourselves to the world, it directs the outcome. This is therefore very pervasive, and we need to be able to understand its role to allow us to grow into our greatness.

In Sports

Team scouts are employed, analytical tools are used as various sports teams search for their next star. Inadvertently, they communicate a fixed mind set doctrine without recognizing it. In a nutshell, they tell us that a person with certain specific attributes will become the star being searched for, falsely telling us that stars are born. As if saying to us that we can do nothing to develop a person into the star we want him or hope that he becomes.

It is not mine to suggest that individuals are born with certain attributes which if cultivated and appropriately nourished will allow them to blossom to eventually become stars. In fact, if we review the parable of the talent in chapter 6 above it will be realized that we are all given at least one talent, what happens subsequently defines who we become. In the parable above let us identify the servants numerically. Servant, one got five talents, servant, two got three talents and servant, three got a single talent. They all got a base from which to launch; what happened next, you may agree, was determined by their mindset. Whereas both servants one and two saw this as an opportunity, servant three saw it differently, more as an entity that needed to be protected. The bible in Luke 12:48 says for unto whomsoever much is given, of him shall be much required; John F. Kennedy in more recent times stated it slightly differently for those to whom much is given, much is required. We can all agree that we were all started with the raw material necessary to allow us to grow into our excellence. Albeit we were given different portions. So, we will not all become businessmen, nor politicians, nor lawyers, nor doctors, but that which we are given is enough seed to allow us to grow into our excellence. We can either choose to cultivate it or bury it. The choice is always ours. If we believe that we have been gifted all that we need, then we would be catering to a fixed mindset and by failing to nurture it, we would be effectively burying it. This attitude with its pervasive tentacles will infiltrate and affect every aspect of our lives. If though we recognize the value of developing what we were gifted through commitment, belief, hard work, and the acknowledgement of support from others, we would be catering to a growth mindset which with its tentacles is able to affect all aspects of our lives.

With a fixed mindset the first challenge presented to that individual may evoke a crisis and have him questioning whether what he has been told all along was true and to address that dilemma, he may either try to explain it away or blame something or someone or alternatively he may just sink into depression because of his interpretation of a challenge as a failure. Let's visit the effect of this mindset on two well-known sports men and the reaction to challenges.

Firstly, the great Tennis player John McEnroe. John was among the greatest players of his time. He may unfortunately be better remembered for his on-court tantrums and eagerness to blame and find excuses for his failures. Compare the attitude of John to another sporting great, this time in the sport of basketball, Michael Jordan. Michael was not considered good enough to make his high school basketball team. He saw this as a challenge and his mother instead of pitying him and trying to win his affection, did not say to him maybe the coach did not like him but instead she offered him constructive advice, "get in the Gym and work harder". In essence she said to him you have the raw material go out and develop it. The rest, as is commonly said, is history. He became one of the greatest basketball players of all time. In his induction to the Naismith basketball hall of fame speech, he recalled the challenges that he experienced during his development as tantamount to wood being added to fire. For him these challenges were not meant to diminish him but to overcome to allow him to shine more brightly. A mind set which allowed him to grow into excellence. He recalls that he has missed more than 9, 9,000 and shots in his career, he has lost over 300 games and twenty -six times he had been trusted to take the game winning shot and missed. Yet he kept going, seeing every hurdle in the eyes of his mother's advice, 'Get in the Gym and work harder, a concept he bought into and in the end he summed it up quite nicely by indicating that he became who he was through hard work, perseverance and the right attitude. For those of us observing his journey, we saw him grow into excellence by employing the BMS Ecosystem. Had he believed that he was a natural which clearly, he was not, we would not be learning about him today. Had his mother evoked the view that he was gifted and did not need to work at his craft, he would not have grown into his excellence to allow us to talk and learn about him and the value of a growth mindset.

Character versus Mindset

The story books are replete with stories of hero's and how they acquired the tag, Jackie Joyner-Kersee, the famed American decathlon athlete in one of her victories had to talk herself through an asthmatic attack to secure a victory. The significance of this is best appreciated when it is realized that exercise can induce an asthmatic attack. Similarly, Pete Sampras, the tennis player of 2000, whilst chasing Roy Emerson's record, was on the brink of defeat at the hands of the younger Patrick Rafter. He was one set down and not playing his best tennis but still was able to emerge victorious. When asked how he did it, he looked for a frame of reference and simply recalled similar scenarios when he was able to pull through. The commentators after the game commented that Sampras returned from the brink of defeat and displayed the qualities of a hero to emerge victorious.

Most would argue that this reflected the character, will and the mind of a champion. What is this? You ask. All of this reflects the growth mindset. It is that uneasiness that makes you practice, it is what allows you to dig down deep and pull it out when you most need it. Does it therefore mean that with that ability you should always be at the top of your game?

Staying on Top

We have noted that athletes like Mike Tyson and Martina Hingis reached the top but did not remain at the top and you ask why? John Wooden, the famed basketball coach, believes that it takes ability to take you to the top but character to keep you there. One gets to the top and assumes that he or she is sufficiently great to just show up without preparation to maintain his/her dominance. It quickly dawns on those who will listen that it takes real character to keep working as hard or even harder to maintain your position. Lessons can be learned from Floyd 'Money' Mayweather who despite his lavish lifestyle valued the importance of doing what it took to prepare himself before a fight. He retired with 50 wins and undefeated in a boxing career spanning 21 years.

Success versus Failure – A Mindset Perspective

As intimated above, there are two different mindsets, a fixed mindset, and a growth mindset. People with a growth mindset tend to focus on process, since they find success in learning and improving. For example, Jackie Joyner-Kersee claimed that she derived just as much happiness from the process as well as the result. She claims she did not mind losing if she saw improvements, or she gave of her best.

Essentially, these athletes with a growth mindset found setbacks motivating. They allowed them introspection, much like a wake-up call.

For those with a fixed mind set success seems a revalidation exercise. Proof that they are superior. In people with a fixed mindset, effort is not cause for pride. People with the growth mindset seem to enjoy the process, those with a fixed mindset, do not subscribe to the need to expend effort to grow into their excellence. Failure fails to motivate the fixed mindset individual, it embarrasses them. They seek to rationalize their failure with excuses or by blaming outside forces.

Mindset and Team Dynamics

What is the role of a star on a team? Maybe, some will argue to be great and win games, occasionally though, a star takes over and wins a game, but a series is more often won by a team.

In the fixed mindset, athletes will want to validate their talent. This may lead to them developing some behavioral issues designed to validate them, seemingly, acting superior to their other teammates, not just a team member. This therefore tends to work against the team concept of together each will achieve more. It appears that in persons with a fixed mindset there is the ongoing struggle coined into the syndrome, the somebody-nobody syndrome. Essentially if I win, I will be somebody. If I lose, I will be nobody. There is an ongoing need for validation which would mean protecting themselves from losing.

Mindset in Business and Leadership

As stated in the title of this chapter, mindset has its tentacles pervading all aspects of our life and can be seen even in business and leadership.

In 2001, when the American company Enron failed, the new yorker writer, Malcolm Gladwell, lamented that it was a result of mindset, claiming that American companies had been obsessed with talent. The primer management consulting firm in the country were insisting that corporate success required the talent mind set. They likened their belief to claiming that there are naturals in sports and so too there are naturals in business. They believed that no expense should be spared in recruiting the best talent. They believed that talent was the key to beating their competition. We have seen above that Talent is akin to a fixed mind set. After paying huge sums to attract what they considered to be talent, they encouraged the development of a fixed mind-set by adoring their talented individuals, which caused their employees to look and act the part, that is seem extraordinarily talented. Research tells us about people with this mindset will do anything, including lying. Integral was the type of leader to make a flaw tolerable. With this mind, setting remedial courses to correct flaws are never explored.

Jim Collins embarked on a five-year study to determine the blueprint that allowed companies to leap from good to great. He selected 11 companies which were able to sustain their edge for a minimum of fifteen years.

He concluded that there were several important factors, but one which he considered was essential was the type of its leader. He described the leaders of those companies as not the larger-than-life charismatic types who oozed ego and self-proclaimed talent. Instead, he found self-effacing people who constantly asked questions and had the ability to confront the most brutal answers. Accepting failures but maintaining faith that they will succeed. These leaders had the hallmark of the growth mind-set. They believed in human development. Pecking order does not seem relevant in this business, individuals are credited for their contributions and the need to undermine others to feel powerful does not seem to exist. These companies explore their own mistakes and shortcomings and seek to engage skills that they and the company will need in the future. With this they grow on templates based on facts not on the fantasy of talent.

The case of Alan Wurtzel is notable, as CEO of the electronic chain, circuit city, he took a company from the brink of bankruptcy and in fifteen years this same company was delivering the highest total return to its stockholders of any firm on the New York stock exchange.

It is important to note that fixed mindset leaders of companies in general mirror fixed mindset people and in these establishments some people are superior, others are treated as inferior. This feeling must be stroked, so the company becomes a simple platform for this. In the companies in which leaders were perceived to have a fixed mind set, the leaders seemingly had a large personal ego which in a large part hastened the company's demise or stagnated its growth. These companies seemed to have a structure akin to a genius with a thousand helpers as opposed to building a great management team. It is striking to note that in none of the autobiographies of the fixed mindset leaders was there any hint of an employee development program. This is the opposite in companies led by leaders with a growth mind set.

ORGANIZATIONAL MINDSET

Can organizations have a mindset? Can the organization's belief be that talent is fixed or that it can be developed? How does the attempt at developing talent in an organization affect the organization? Based on work done by Dr Dweck, we have come to recognize two different organizational cultures which mirror the organizational mindset. The culture of genius, seen in a fixed organizational mindset and the culture of development which is seen in the growth organizational mindset. The impact of these mindsets on the employees is telling; people in the growth mindset organization seem to have much more trust in their company, a much greater sense of empowerment, ownership, and commitment. Interestingly, those who worked in fixed mindset companies were more eager to leave their company for another.

Our learning of mindsets and behavior thus far recognizes that with a fixed mindset the tendency is for one to show that he/she is of a superior ilk, his behaviors either knowingly or not is rooted in the need to prove himself or herself this however has a trickle-down effect with the employees more likely to hide information and malign their colleagues in an effort to look or feel superior.

Does Mindset Affect Relationships?

We have commented above on the pervasive nature of mindset, so the obvious question is does mindset have a role in relationships? If as we contend that mindset is very pervasive and with its tentacles invades every aspect of human beings; let's see if it influences intimate relationships. We have heard repeatedly that in an effort to sustain relationships we need to work on them, is that a hint of mindset coming to the fore?

We have also seen a variety of behaviors brought on by failed relationships, so one wonders what role if any does mindset play in a relationship and are there any repercussions attributable to mindset that causes a relationship to fail or succeed.

I have seen at least two acquaintances of mine suffer severely from failed relationships both requiring psychiatric support following such an event. We know of the broken heart syndrome addressed in my book on cardiovascular disease; a condition precipitated by stress. So, we know that stress contributes to the outcome of any failed relationship, giving an organic element to the impact of a failed relationship. And Interestingly, research shows that people with a fixed mindset felt judged or labeled by the failed relationship. It felt that everyone who met them through some invisible means thought that they were unlovable, so they evoked an invisible barrier around their person. There was almost a universal desire to neutralize that pain of rejection by hurting the person who hurt them, a sort of blame and punish tendency. Typical of the fixed mindset, the cause for their discomfort is always external to them. There is a willingness to find an excuse, to blame and even to punish. This seems to be a thread which is common to individuals with fixed mindsets. The attempt at self-protection, but does mindset also contribute?

With people with a growth mindset the approach was different, it was more an act of understanding, forgiving, learning, and moving on with their lives. In essence every relationship screams for a growth mindset, since it teaches you who is right for you. The two acquaintances of mine who needed psychological support following the termination of a relationship were obviously of a fixed mindset. They found it difficult to forgive and forget. Individuals with a growth mindset learnt from the experience and instead of living in the past, they could put the experience behind them and look to the future having learnt from that experience. Daniel Goleman in his expose' on emotional intelligence; remarks social-emotional skills, I can tell you what they are, but mindsets add another dimension. They help us understand why people don't learn the skills they need or use the skills they have.

With a fixed mindset, falling in love introduces at least two other variants, (a) The mindset of your partner and (b) your mindset towards the relationship. You see with a fixed mindset, you believe that your character traits are fixed and can't be changed, the same for your partner and the relationship, so there is no appetite to work on the relationship. With a fixed mindset, the caste system is invariably evoked. Who is the superior entity? Who is better, more talented than who? Will the relationship be developed any further? Was this relationship meant to be or not? How does the relationship deal with challenges? The response to these questions is based on judgement.

In a growth mindset, we know that your traits can be developed, so too your partner's and not least the relationship. It therefore requires work.

Analyzing relationships with people with a fixed mindset, one immediately foresees two issues. In the fixed mindset, the expectation is that everything good will happen automatically. It in no way suggests a desire for the components of this partnership to work to help each other solve their problems or gain skills. There is this belief that this should happen magically through their professed love. You may have heard statements of the type: my partner should know what I think, feel, and need and vice versa. This is not only ridiculous, but also impossible; more like a figment of one's imagination. The second issue is that with a fixed mindset and problem, which are inevitable in a relationship, may be seen as a sign of flaws in the relationship. People with a fixed mindset talk about problems in their relationship by usually assigning blame. Rarely do they blame themselves, but more usually they blame the partner. The blame is usually in relation to a particular trait of the partner, a character flaw.

In people with a fixed mindset in relationships the role of the other party oscillates, one moment he is an ally the best thing that could be dreamt of, another moment he is the enemy. The relationship may also serve as a segway allowing you to divert attention from yourself. When you fail at a task, it's hard to continue to blame someone else but in a relationship, there is the other person who can be blamed.

In the fixed mindset there is always the need for self-affirmation so competition to show you up as the greater character, a feature most would agree which should have no place in a relationship, becomes almost inevitable.

In embarking unto a relationship, there are two characters with different traits, in a growth mindset, it is advisable that both parties develop the skills necessary to deal with the traits from their partner, with this approach both partners grow, and the relationship deepens.

There is clear evidence that mindset does not only affect and guide the behavior of the individual, but it infiltrates his entire interaction with society. So, if we consider mindset as an internal construct, it is sufficiently pervasive to spread its tentacles to affect every aspect of the person's existence, including how we present ourselves to the public and their perception of us.

In developing friendships, we are given an opportunity to both enhance and validate each other. This may necessitate the issuance of praise and sometimes we need reassurance about ourselves. These occasions can be used to provide support as well as relaying a message of growth. In the fixed mindset, the need to prove yourself may arise with a detrimental effect on the friendship. To the person with the fixed mindset there is an ongoing need for self-validation, the lower a person is the better you may feel.

Could this lead to individuals becoming shy? Shy people may consciously or unconsciously worry that others may embarrass or judge them in social settings. Shy people with a fixed mindset may exhibit a host of features which clearly indicate fear. It is not uncommon for them to exhibit anxiety, experience heart racing, avoiding eye contact etc., all features of a desire to escape the setting quickly. It has been shown that shyness harms the social interaction with people with a fixed mindset but not those with a growth mindset. You may wonder why and how people considered shy behave differently in the same social setting.

People with a growth mind set may still be considered shy and experience the same uneasiness in a social setting. Those with a growth mindset though will consider the social setting a new challenge, so although they feel anxious, they will welcome the opportunity to meet someone new. The fixed and growth mindset people approached the identical situation with different attitudes; the growth mindset people feel less shy and nervous as the interaction continues in other words, they embrace the experience while the fixed mindset people fear the experience and rarely, if ever, become comfortable.

We spoke of shyness what of bullies, does mindset play a role?

You would have realized thus far that people with a fixed mindset need constant validation. How better to ensure your validation than being a bully. Bullying is about judging, the more powerful kids judging the less powerful kids. Here a fixed mind set works both ways (1) the need to be superior and hence validate yourself by bullying someone clearly does the job. The person being bullied if he also has a fixed mindset feels diminished and he may choose to elevate his standing by lashing out. Think of the number of school shootings we have heard about and the common association with bullying. However, once the person who is bullied stands up against the bully and either defeats him or neutralizes his antics, he never bully's that individual again. Why may you ask? Could it be his perceived superiority has been challenged and he is now forced to second guess himself that he is no longer who he thought he was. Remember fixed mindsets never deal well with challenges.

Reflection:

Are we guilty as a society for the creation of mindsets?

Can one only get by on talent?

During scouting exercises what do scouts look for Talent or work ethic

Does one character arise from his/her mindset?

What does one require to remain at the top of his/her game?

Does one's mindset determine how he/she deals with failure?

Does mindset determine team dynamics?

Does the functioning of a team reflect the mindset of its leader?

Can a business reflect the mindset of its leader?

Does mindset determine how one responds to success?

Is an organization likely to mirror the mindset of its boss?

Does an organizational mindset influence the relationship between its employees?

_____

_____

_____

_____

_____

_____

_____

_____

_____

_____

_____

Chapter 9: The Birth and Cultivation of Mindsets

"It's not that I am so smart, it's just that I stay with problems longer." —
Albert Einstein

The Beginnings

We have spoken ad nauseum about mindsets, but where does it
come from? How is it cultivated?

Most would tell us that at birth we have the blueprints for the
potential of whom we may become but with the interaction with our
environment we morph into who we eventually become. I am not saying
that we are born with distinctive mindsets, I am just contending that we
have the rudimentary trappings of a mindset which is allowed to blossom
into a growth or fixed mindset as we interact with our environment.

We recognize that from infancy, the newborn quickly understands
what types of behaviors they must exhibit if they are to provoke a
particular response.

When they are hungry, they cry until they are fed, if they are wet
or soiled, they will cry so, the practice is continued. One may quickly
intervene to claim that this is the only recourse for the newborn. But that
is not very accurate, had we not responded to the cries of the newborn,
he/she would no longer cry when hungry, a type of learned or condition
reflex much like Pavlov experiments on salivation with dogs.

In a similar manner, as memorialized in the poem by Dorothy Law Nolte, Children learn what they live. We can start imagining that since our parents are our first teachers the buds of mindset begin to develop in our early years as our parents' massage various aspects of our being.

Parents generally, maybe, innocently, are willing to do or give anything that they believe will help their children feel better and make them successful.

Children, we have been told, are like sponges absorbing what is said to them or done to and for them. Every word and action send a message to the children. It tells them how to think about themselves or gives them an indication of how they are perceived initially by their parents who supposedly love them and supposedly know them best.

It may be the germination of a fixed mindset, that sort of tells the child that she has permanent traits which are being judged by her parents. Am I saying that we should not praise our children. Praise may either encourage the development of a fixed mindset or a growth mindset. By praising ability, we signal to the child that he/she has some special fixed innate quality. On the other hand, by praising the process and acknowledging the effort put in by the youngster, you are effectively helping him to appreciate the value of effort in obtaining results. Seeds which lead to the development of a growth mindset.

Remember children are very sensitive and the message they hear from a comment may not have been what you intended.

Telling Melissa, she is smart and coating it with apparent evidence causes her to believe you. For example, if you say to Melissa, she is smart, as evidence of her smartness she got through her work quickly, or she scored an A without even studying because she is real smart. Melissa interprets this to mean that if she does not complete her work quickly, she is not smart. If she must study, it means that she is not smart. To maintain that label, she does minimal studying and simultaneously rushes through her work with the hope of maintaining the semblance of smartness. This generates a behavioral pattern in Melissa which would be governed by a fixed mindset. Teachers may also be guilty of the same practice and sayings, leading to concretization of the fixed mindset.

So, should we not praise our children? What must we say to encourage our children? How do we encourage confidence in them? How do we compliment them on their achievements?

The reaction of children to praise leaves no doubt that children love praise, so are we to deprive them of those little things that they love? And which we do to encourage the development of their confidence and abilities?

Allow me to share a father-son experience between my father and Myself with you.

As a young adult, one day after playing cricket and batting for virtually the entire day without losing my wicket; when I returned home my father looked me straight in the eye and said a few words to me which I have held on too since that time. He said, "Son, whatever you put your mind too, you seem to be above average". You may not believe but I have held onto those words and cherished them till today. The message I got from his statement is that I have the tools and if I put my mind (commit) to any task, as per his observation, the results are better than average. Commitment requires discipline and work to be ready for any task on which you will embark. These words continue to be the extra push that I have fallen back on whenever I am faced with a challenge. It clearly shows how my father instilled a growth mind set in me. Encapsulated in his message is the need to commit, once that is done your results will be better than average. You may wonder what I understood by putting my mind to the task. By putting my mind to the task, it talks to commitment. With commitment, the question is asked, what do you need to do to show that you have committed yourself to the task. Commitment requires dedication and dedication requires work to develop and maintain your skill set. It is a process and to hear the individual who knew me best, my father, tell me in essence that to achieve, a process is involved and if I commit, I will do better than my average competition. Fewer words have meant more to me than those. Those were not the only words my father said to me but those were the ones that got stuck in my memory, why? you may ask. I believe it was because of the impact these words had on me. I still rely on these words even today, some twenty-eight years since my father departed from this life. We must be careful with the words that we use to our children and the messages we communicate. Surely, children can be irritating and can cause you to get annoyed but as adults what we say to children is a major contributor to the development of their mindset, which as we have seen is pervasive and influences every aspect of their lives.

Addressing Failure

Failure is a greater more delicate issue to address, the child will most likely be upset and already discouraged by the failure.

Not long ago I read a story of this nine-year-old who was about to enter her first gymnastics competition. She had all the attributes which were ideally suited to a gymnast. She was confident that she would win the competition. She had even pictured where she would place the trophy in her room.

Unfortunately, the competition took place, but she won nothing and she was broken, deflated and devastated.

As a parent how does one approach her, recognizing that you could damage her confidence for life.

A. Do you tell her she was the best?

B. Tell her the judges did not like her, so they robbed her.

C. Try to pacify her and get her mind, albeit temporarily, off the event by telling her that gymnastics is not important and there are numerous other activities at which she is good.

D. Tell her that she has the ability and with a different Judge she will surely win next time.

E. Tell her that she is just not good enough!

The societal message of protecting and boosting children self-esteem is to protect them from failure.

A. If you as a parent opted for the first reaction, you would effectively mislead.

B. In the second reaction you are apportioning blame, a feature of the fixed mindset.

C. The third reaction suggests a type of attitude that encourages her to devalue an activity or event if she fails to do well.

D. To tell her that she has the ability, although it may be so, sends the dangerous message that if she believes that she has the ability, then she should win, but one may argue, does it not lay the template for a greater lesson?

E. The final reaction that she is not good enough, though superficially appearing heartless, may offer the best opportunity for profound learning. Her father told her exactly that, he first empathized with her he acknowledged that she did her best and recognized how that must have made her feel. Now the blow was more digestible, telling her she had not really earn it yet. He helped her to understand that to become a winner she had to work harder and get better. The message *if that is something she really wants, she would have to work harder.* She understood that if she wanted to do gymnastics as a recreational sport, that would be okay, but if she wanted to be a champion, she would have to work harder.

The young child got the message, and she went back to the drawing board, improved her skill set and at the next meeting, she was crowned the overall champion.

The value of this story is that children don't need protection, they need honesty. Withholding constructive criticism does not help children's confidence as in the case above it led to an improved product.

Is Discipline Teaching?

In my part of the world when children annoy their parents sufficiently, you may hear statements, prior to the imposition of punishment as I will teach you a lesson you will never forget; and many simply go along with this, but is this really teaching? And if so what lesson is being taught?

Though it may not be manifestly obvious, the children may be understanding that if they go against their parents' wishes, they will be judged and punished. These children are not being taught how to think through the issues and make a mature decision.

The roles of parents, teachers and coaches are crucially important, as are the words they use and the messages they communicate in shaping future generations. We have spoken about the need for praising our children, yet we have said praise is a crucial component in the development of the mindset. We know of two mindsets. A fixed mindset and a growth mindset, we have seen the type of praise which encourages the development of the fixed mindset. Is there any type of praise which encourages the development of a growth mindset?

You will recall that above the praise to the children was based on their intelligence, not their effort, this practice, though not intentional, has a sinister effect on the children. It leads them into a mindset which requires ongoing validation. It also erodes their confidence, causing them

103

to shy away from any task which challenges the belief that we, parents, teachers, and coaches sewed and cultivated.

Instead of praising our children for some innate ability, we should seek more to praise them for their effort, their persistence and somehow link the outcome to that process. This has the ability for developing a mindset in which children begin to appreciate the challenge and it may lead to the blossoming of the growth mindset. Praise is more effective in the development of the growth mindset when the focus is on the process and the effort expended rather than only on the result and some innate ability, such as talent, which brought the desired result to the fore.

Be careful with our words, by praising our children for their efforts but by showing our disgust to the achievements or non-achievements of our neighbors children, through our chosen words, like nothing better is expected of Tom because he is a born failure, or he is an air head, or you may gloat in someone's successes by talking about their talent and aptitude with expressions like Jessie is a born genius, I wish she was my daughter. It may lead to the germination and cultivation of a fixed mindset. One must therefore be careful; success can drive you into a fixed mindset.

Is there a False Growth Mindset?

We have been addressing mindset repeatedly as separate, distinct, entities insinuating that an individual either has a positive or negative mindset, it is without doubt that both mindsets coexist in the same individual, and the mindset with which we operate oscillate from time to time. If we can appreciate the nature of both mindsets, we will be able to identify the dominant mindset with which we operate. We will also be able to determine when a fixed mindset is being triggered and in the next section, we will inform how we can change from a fixed to a growth mindset.

Some people may mistakenly see themselves as having a growth mindset because they are open-minded or flexible. With a growth mindset, though there is need for evidence of effort to ensure change. So, if you are open minded but show no desire, or make no effort for developing yourself or others, it would argue against a growth mindset. Open mindedness is not equivalent to a growth mindset. A growth mindset assesses two major elements effort and results. If you claim to be putting in effort but the results are not commensurate, it may not be that the individual is operating from a growth mindset. One may have great results but little to no effort been expended, though this would suggest the development of a growth mindset, it does not approach a growth mindset. A growth mindset always marries effort with results.

Since we recognize the prominence of effort in the growth mindset, there is this misconception that effort is all there is to define the growth mindset. We have pointed out the importance of praising effort in the development of a growth mindset in children and tying it to the results. Simultaneously, efforts without results could reflect an incorrect approach. We love to recognize the process, the effort, method, and the results. So, effort is not the only requirement to define a growth mindset, it is an integral component though. Praising effort, which is not present, does not encourage the development of the growth mindset.

It may be true that children can do anything but by telling them that do not engineer some magical conversion. It is more likely to happen if you encourage and facilitate the development of the requisite skills. Though you may encourage and even facilitate the acquisition of the requisite skill, the onus is still on the person who you hope will develop the growth mindset to acquire the proposed goal. In this scenario, the person may be adjudged as a failure, since he/she has failed to achieve the desired goal, but the question becomes was the role of the tutor appropriately executed or was the environment sufficiently growth mindset appealing in which individuals feel safe and free from being judged. Finally, our words, claiming that we have a growth mindset does not always coalesce with our actions. Hence either creating confusion or frustration with the communicated message.

Reflection

What gives rise to mindset?

Do we participate in its creation inadvertently?

When we discipline children, are we teaching?

Is there an entity called a false growth mindset?

Are you guilty of believing that you have a growth mindset when your actions and thoughts are that of a fixed mindset?

How is failure addressed by you?

Are you more likely to try to explain your failures or blame something or someone for your failure?

Do failures allow you to grow?

_____

_____

_____

_____

_____

_____

_____

_____

Chapter 10: Nourishment of the Mind

"Nourish your mind like you would your body. The mind cannot survive on junk food". — Jim Rohn

Not Discernable by Our Senses

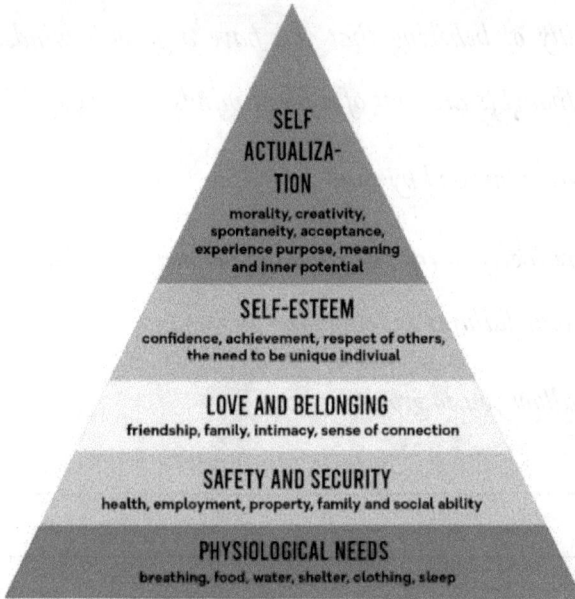

Let's go back to visit Maslow's hierarchy of needs. As we understand each level of the pyramid must be fully attended to before you can continue to move up to a higher round, and finally to the top, which is "Self-Actualization". You have fully attended to your physiological needs, so now we must go on to your mind.

Again and again in this modern era, we can no longer regard good health as just 'the absence of illnesses. With the emergence of positive psychology, evidence is unfolding that positive thinking is good for physical health, mental health, relationships, and performance in all aspects of life. Unfortunately, there is no one plaster solution to negative mindset, nor is there a magic wand to wave to convert a negative mindset to a positive mindset. The change from having a negative mindset to a positive mindset is a process which requires time and effort. The change is worth the effort for a negative mindset individual sees difficulty with every opportunity while a positive mindset individual sees the opportunity in every difficulty.

When addressing nourishing of the mind we are not talking about eating vegan and ensuring you are drinking enough water. It has nothing to do with what you put in your mouth. Because we are referring to the mind, I will be discussing what you put into your mind, your belief systems, and your thoughts. Afterall, your thoughts are the foundation of your belief system. You must remember that "truths" to you are nothing but beliefs which you hold on to, and these beliefs guide your thoughts and contribute to your mindset.

Fixed Mindset and Growth Mindset

Your thought processes create a basis for nourishment of the mind. Your mind will react appropriately to how we speak to it, and how we speak to it is influenced by our mindset. There are two distinguishable mindsets that are prevalent in people: a fixed mindset and a growth mindset. With a **fixed mindset (as in the story of the talents above, the servant who buried his talent),** the individual believes that their basic abilities, intelligence, and talents are fixed traits. With a **growth**

mindset (again as in the story of the talents above, the servants who doubled their talents), individuals believe that their abilities and intelligence can be developed with effort, learning and ambition. Nourishing your mindset comes down to your mental attitude, be it simply a positive attitude or negative one. It is of utmost importance that you understand the voice of the positive mindset so that you may be able to nourish your mind.

An individual with a fixed mindset is virtually stuck and has no desire for growth or improvement. They believe, as in the story of the talents in chapter 6, that they can only lose, so they avoid challenging themself and aim to remain in their comfort zone.

They blame their shortcomings on their perceived lack of talent and ability. The operative reaction is to always place blame on someone or something else and to never accept responsibility for their life or truly learn (therefore grow) from the challenge. It is not surprising that individuals with a fixed mindset tend to be associated with a negative mental attitude. Reflecting on the Parable of Talents, we see clearly that the third servant who was given one talent had a fixed mindset. When his master questioned him, the servant offered excuses for his failure and was then judged as wicked and lazy. Now, I am not saying that those who have fixed mindsets are wicked and lazy! But by not attempting to grow or explore their potential, they may be considered as such since they are robbing society of the benefit of being exposed to their talents and the achievements that result.

As Albert Einstein said, "Nothing happens until something moves", would it not be safe to call someone lazy because they remain in their comfort zone and failed to move out of their comfort zone? I think it is useful to observe that when one has a fixed mindset one usually doesn't take responsibility for their shortcomings. Again, you remain locked in a cycle governed by a belief system that not only does not serve you, but it can also keep you from happiness and living a fuller life. This way of operating is very different from having a growth mindset.

When one possesses a growth mindset you believe in your abilities and intelligence and are willing to challenge yourself by developing them further. You have a greater drive and will persevere in the face of setbacks. You accept mistakes as small challenges that offer you an opportunity to improve. A growth mindset may be nourished through effort-oriented praise from a leader in your life.

When you possess a growth mindset, you look for opportunities to develop yourself. You readily jump into further education or training based on your needs knowing that you will be better for it in the long run. When you possess a growth mindset you will exude positivity. Your positive energy not only lights you up, but also lights up people around you. You see a situation with a "glass half full" attitude and therefore dedicate yourself to continue growing and taking full responsibility for yourself to make the glass full.

The Repair of a Fixed Mindset and Nourishing a Growth Mindset

Dr Sonja Lyubomirsky's research indicates that 40% of our ability to sustain happiness and positivity is mediated by three skills: (a) Our ability to reframe an experience into a more positive interpretation, (b) our ability to experience gratitude and (c) our choice to be kind and generous. Research clearly shows that the mere shifting of your focus from the negative aspects in your life to more positive ones will promote happiness and well-being.

The more one tries to avoid negative thoughts and feelings the more it impinges on our mental space even against our wishes. Unfortunately, throughout our growth we are primed to focus more on the negative than the positive. It is believed that this is a survival trait that we have learnt, or it may be the exercise of the ego trying to protect us. Luckily, we can learn to shift our focus from negative to positive.

You may now be asking yourself how can one repair or convert a fixed mindset into a growth mindset, especially if you tend to operate from that place. First recognize and take comfort that a fixed mindset is not always in constant operation and has several triggers. These triggers can look like challenges, setbacks, hard work, criticism, and the success of others. These triggers limit your potential when you are in a fixed mindset as you meet them with defeat and excuses as opposed to the willingness to try harder. A totally different approach to that which we see in a growth mindset. As with so many things in life, you can help yourself and change a fixed mindset.

Here are some manageable steps to fighting back against the fixed mindset within yourself:

Be willing to learn your fixed mind set voice and engage it in conversation.

I'm sure you have had an experience where you think of trying something new but immediately, you start having thoughts of why it should or should not be done. The fixed mindset will encourage you to remain in your comfort zone, while your growth mindset will encourage you to see ways in which it can be done. Even if you do not have the skill set, your growth mindset will encourage you to find the help you require to move forward.

If you can identify the voice of your fixed mindset, you can silence it. Remember you always have a choice; you have the choice to move forward. You can avoid the negative thoughts associated with a fixed mindset by creating a mental distraction, and hence silence the voice of the negative mindset. This may require only a few seconds. A physical distraction may also be useful.

Recognize the growth mindset voice and as you engage the fixed mindset in conversation, you must be prepared to employ the growth mindset voice. Finding a positive friend can also be helpful when the negative thoughts of a fixed mindset visits or alternatively you could reflect on associated positives. If you are inundated with the negative thoughts of a fixed mindset, you can snap out of those thoughts by creating a list and then throwing it away. It provides useful distraction and may allow you to reflect on the negative thoughts more deeply. You must be prepared to ask yourself the question "why?" and be willing to reflect on what will happen to you if you listen to your fixed mindset voice or are willing to go forward with your growth mindset.

Once you recognize the growth mindset voice, be prepared to take the growth mindset advice. And its advice is usually simple: "You should do it because it is possible."

You must show gratitude and appreciation for what you have. Put less focus on what you don't have. It does not matter what you're grateful for, how big or small. You may wish to show gratitude by recognizing the role others play in your good fortune and well-being. It allows you to take pleasure in life's small joys. This can help you to focus on the now; and magnetizes your desire allowing you to attract appropriate vibrations and move you up the emotional guidance system (EGS) towards level 1. **N.B** A single expression of gratitude to another person can boost your mood for a month or more. For gratitude to have a long-lasting effect on your daily happiness, it is advisable to incorporate gratitude into your everyday life. Creating a gratitude Journal or letter will greatly facilitate this process.

The Dangers of a Fixed Mindset

People with a fixed mindset have very particular traits and shortcomings. They see challenges in their life as a barrier rather than an opportunity. Because of this, they rarely excel at anything as they would rather invest their energies into looking smart rather than investing in being smart. When the fixed mindset is in the driver's seat you are constantly filled with excuses and blame as opposed to taking responsibility for your own shortcomings. As you can imagine or may have personally experienced, this mindset keeps one stagnant and at a standstill in their life. It virtually keeps you on a treadmill: your

surroundings change but you remain unchanged. It is no wonder why people who constantly allow their minds to have these limits are never pioneers and rarely leaders in this world.

One of my favorite stories that demonstrates the power of overcoming a fixed mindset is that of Sir Roger Gilbert Bannister and his contribution to the sport of long-distance running. Prior to 1954, no human being living, or dead had run a mile in under four minutes, it was the popular view that it was too great a feat for a human being. It was truly thought of as impossible, and the view was that it could not be done. Then, despite this common belief, Roger Bannister ran a sub-four-minute mile in the 1954 Helsinki Olympics. Just knowing this feat was possible dramatically changed many athletes from having a fixed mindset to a growth mindset. Today, over 400 American athletes (including high school students!) have run sub-4-minute miles. Steve Scott, an American middle-distance runner has individually run a sub-4-minute mile 137 times. This exemplifies the power of proper "nourishment" The **IT IS POSSIBLE NOURISHMENT** with which you feed your mind.

In the example of running the sub-4-minute mile the only thing that changed was the belief system. The mile is still the same distance. Athletes are still human beings! Except in 1954, it was proven that it is possible. The belief system and thus the mindset brought forth this change. With this clear example, I am sure you now have many personal moments when your beliefs have tricked you into staying in a fixed mindset. The only way to really revive your mind and ensure you stay on track to living a long and vibrant life is to nourish your growth mindset. Without it you will remain stuck and never realize your full potential.

Reflection:

Based on evidence above, do I generally operate from a growth or fixed mindset?

What three things I can do right now in my life to nourish a growth mindset?

Can I think of someone in my life who has a growth mindset?

What are their defining traits?

_____

_____

_____

_____

_____

_____

_____

_____

What other supports can you employ to continue to nourish your mind? Look at your environment and the respective messages. You can choose to appropriately nourish your mind to facilitate a growth mindset or to hold onto the fixed mindset and continue to blame others for your shortcoming. Now that you are aware of this, your decision becomes informed.

Chapter 11: The Effect of the Environment on Your Mind

"What lies behind you and what lies in front of you, pales in comparison to what lies inside of you." - Ralph Waldo Emerson

The Mind and its Environment

When you wake up in the morning you may have a very clear intention of how you want to approach your day. You may feel confident and ready to take on all the tasks and work at hand. As the day progresses it becomes clear that stimuli designed with ulterior purposes are constantly coming at you, and not all of them are constructive. We live in a world in which most of our influences are negative and so we must actively work to make a change. For example, people may offer well-intentioned advice because they feel it is in your best interest. However, it is coming from their own belief systems. You may come across people who are constantly blaming others or circumstances for their own stagnation.

Be it our own family, co-workers, or strangers with whom we cross paths, the people that surround us can create a corrosive and negative environment in which it is a struggle to nurture our mind in positive ways. Let us examine some ways in which you can keep your surroundings more positive which will feed into your inspiration and nurture a growth mindset.

Neutralizing a Hostile Environment

Understanding how to neutralize the negativity that surrounds you is an essential skill if you wish to continue reviving your mind and stay on the path to realizing your full potential and living a life full of vitality as you grow into your excellence. Again, I cannot stress enough that if your body is adequately catered to, but your mind suffers, you cannot have access to adding years to our life and life to our years or grow into your excellence. All the parts of your person (the body, mind and spirit) are interconnected.

Some may suggest that you just simply ignore the negativity and go on with your day. However, that is easier said than done! No matter your efforts, some of the adverse chatter will always get through to you.

First, I recommend that you clarify your priorities in life. Perhaps it is to follow through on some important goals or remain very present so that you can create some new goals. When you have a clear idea of what your priorities are you can then work on removing clutter from your life that interferes with your ability to reach these goals. This will include identifying people in your life with fixed mindsets and work on creating distance or removing them all together from your environment, this may include reducing the time spent around them or eliminating them from your core group of associates. Even if they are relatives of yours, You must be prepared to walk away.

Of course, some of these people may be family and friends. You must be willing to manage a bit of emotional fallout if you remove yourself from particular social circles that no longer serve the growth of a more positive mind. Criticism may be directed at you for a change in your behavior, but again you must work on ensuring that the naysayers do not infiltrate your thought processes and belief systems. Stay grounded and strong knowing that you are creating the best life you can for yourself.

I am not recommending that you become asocial, human beings are sociable, I am just suggesting that you become more selective in choosing your friends and associates. Perhaps you may choose to have different categories of associates. For example, there may be some people who you may choose to share a joke or play games with, but from whom you will not seek guidance or advice. You have come to realize that they have negative mindsets, and their contribution will not nourish your mindset and provide it with the appropriate environment in which to blossom. It is about understanding your relationships and the ones that appropriately feed you.

Nourishing "Food" for the Mind

Your mind is nourished by the thoughts that are a product of your mindset. Cultivating your growth mindset is a dynamic daily undertaking, and the process is facilitated by the nourishment you provide. This nourishment is your thoughts, which create the environment in which you allow your mindset to develop.

When beginning your day there are some simple steps to employ to start it on the right footing:

- **Positive affirmations:** This is positive self-talk in which you continuously encourage yourself to see the glass as half full rather than half empty.

120

- **Instill in your belief system that everything is possible:** This will cultivate a new thought pattern so when you are confronted with a challenge, you no longer will say to yourself that it is impossible. Instead, you will remember that it *is* possible and immediately start thinking of ways in which you may overcome the challenge. Whether you choose to go through the challenge or around the challenge, believe you me there is always a way to overcome it!

- **Understand and recognize that no one person knows it all:** This includes you. Yes, sometimes it requires tapping into the expertise of others. Be prepared to learn! Appreciate the value of mentorship and remember that everything is possible!

- **Challenges or negativity will cross your path:** Be prepared to recognize them, confront them, and manage them while keeping a positive attitude throughout your day. Even when you don't feel ready for the challenges, you can get through them! Try.

As you go about your business, always make a commitment to remain neutral in situations or to leave an environment more positive than before you entered it. Create a strong focus on positive experiences no matter how small they are. This commitment to constantly connect to the brightness of your day feeds the growth mindset.

Having a sense of humor is a must! Not only will it further safeguard you from the negativity you will encounter, but it will also strengthen your will when you are faced with your own challenges throughout the day. It will help you escape from negative moments. You will always be confronted with your own failures and shortcomings, but you will be more willing to learn from them. Never forget each failure is an opportunity for learning and supporting your growth mindset and is a step closer to your desired goal.

Continue to focus on the present. The past is gone and cannot be undone. We can never change what has happened in our lives. All we can control is how we react to the present and the choices we make. This is most important in nurturing your mind in a positive way. Connect with the now, as it is all you have.

My Story

Throughout this chapter, we have lamented the volume of negativity which surrounds us daily. Our parents, our siblings, our schoolteachers, and those who we come across in our day-to-day activities. Their negativity seems to be conspiring against us, ensuring that the sinister plot of discouraging us from dreaming or moving from our comfort zones is maintained. In fact, many believe that the cemetery is the wealthiest place on the planet, since within it lies the frustrated dreams, the unwritten New York Times best sellers, the undeveloped potential invention which the conspirators have been able to silence and rob the world from ever experiencing.

Again and again, we have got to find some way of shutting out the chatter. Had the Wright brothers been swayed by the negativism of the day, they would have never developed and flew the first airplane, an invention which you will agree has succeed figuratively in making the world smaller; Had Alexander Graham Bell listened to the distracting noises, he would have never succeeded in pioneering the development of our telephone system, an invention, you will agree, which has succeeded in bringing us together even if we are apart. Had Eric Yuan been guided by the naysayers, his development of Zoom video conferencing software, would have never occurred and the world would have been robbed of this much needed tool for communication which proved priceless during the Covid-19 (coronavirus) pandemic. Thus, giving new meaning to the apparent hitherto meaningless phrase "apart but still together". The world continues to benefit from the efforts of those who filter out the naysayers and allow them to have a limited impact on their activities.

I have been exposed to my fair share of naysayers and I have tried a myriad of ways to avoid the noise. Try as we may there is some noise that tends to get through. This noise may be very damaging with a long-lasting impact. I want to share two such examples from my own life with you of brief statements which were made to me during my teenage years which have had a profound impact on me and the way in which my life has unfolded.

At high school in year 10 I worked hard at my academics as I always did. My overall year position was second among all year 10 students at my school. My form Mistress at the time, in her comments on my report card wrote: 'Harris has the ability but prides himself as the clown of the class'. The teacher was our history teacher, a trusted and respected influence. I had scored an A+ in history during that semester, but that did not matter much; I had forgotten much of what I learnt in her classes, but these comments lived with me; the damage had been done. I loved comedy and loved to ensure that the people with whom I interacted were happy or at least laughing. In fact, looking back, I could have possibly explored comedy as a career. From that comment, I thought comedy was a bad thing, the language used, 'clown' shattered any prospect of me pursuing comedy as a career, the damage was done. It discouraged the development of my comedic skills. The result, the world of comedy and the planet has essentially lost a willing comedian.

Equally important is the noise or chatter that knowingly or unknowingly has a positive impact. During my teenage years, I must admit that I was not particularly focused on any specific career path. Academically, I performed creditably but I also had a keen interest in sports, specifically cricket. In fact, I made the national under 19 trials in cricket in two successive years, one year as an opening batsman and wicket keeper and the second year as a spin bowler and number 3 batsman. I was reasonably okay. I also dabbled in chicken farming and through my methods, my chief and better-established competitor sold all his birds to me and closed his chicken farm.

In the dynamic phase of my teenage years, whilst returning home from a cricket game in which I scored a lot of runs and batted throughout the day without the loss of my wicket. My eldest brother who was a spectator at the games got home before me and told our parents about my performance. On reaching home, my father took a long hard, almost piecing look at me and said, 'Son, it seems that whatever you put your mind too, you are better than average'. I don't know the intention of that statement, but it was not a frivolous comment. I have held onto that statement dearly through the years. I gain both solace and fight from it.

Based on the belief that my father knew me better than any other person living or dead, made that observation, I have believed it, and it has helped me.

Granted my father departed this life about three decades ago but his words have been held sacred by me and continue to live within me. Whenever I am faced with a challenge, that may seem insurmountable, I reflect on those words to spur me forward. I remind myself that since my father knew me better than most will ever know me, and he thinks that I am better than average, then I am not average. This has the invisible power of granting me the 'can do' aura which has helped me to both consciously and unconsciously put a bit more effort into it, knowing that I am better than average. With this mantra I have overcome countless challenges, irrespective of the effort required.

So, you see a kind word can move you forward, allowing you to climb high hills trying to get home. A harsh word, on the other hand, is like a dagger, killing dreams and flushing them to the cemetery which Myles Munroe considers to be the wealthiest place on the planet.

As much as possible surround yourself with others who are dedicated to living their life with a growth mindset. Cultivate friendships with more positive people who understand the importance of nourishing the mind in a positive manner and are on board not only to put these practices in place themselves but are also there to support you. If possible, you may want to change work environments as well. Working on a team or in an office where people are in line with your values can be a game changer. Ideally surrounding yourself with people who have achieved what you seek is among the strongest contributor to the attainment of your goal.

Reflection:

When have I come into a negative environment and had to work on staying positive?

How did it make me feel?

Are there any specific environments in my life that I feel promote a fixed mindset as opposed to nourishing a growth mindset?

What is something I can commit to doing every day to help myself nourish a growth mindset?

_____

_____

_____

_____

_____

_____

_____

_____

_____

_____

We have examined factors which nourish your mind. As you can see, sometimes it can be grand but at other times it can be a subtle word from someone you respect and believe. It depends on your mindset and where you are in the day so that you can make the best decisions. Also, keep in mind that each day is different, and your process may have to change daily depending on what is happening in your life. But I know with practice and dedication you will be able to surmount the challenges you will face. Again, it is all about taking responsibility and to be willing to stay on the course.

To ensure you have a complete set of tools that will allow your growth mindset to flourish, let's dig into aspects of our lives which negatively impact our minds. It is always important to study the insightful and the dull so that you can empower yourself to make the best and most informed choices in reviving your mind, and grow into your excellence .

Chapter 12: Impacting the Mind

"I have learned over the years that when one's mind is made up, this diminishes fear; knowing what must be done does away with fear." – *Rosa Parks*

The Mind

There are varying views on how your mind functions in your life. Some view it purely as a task-based mechanism that runs on its own, while some view it as relatively labile, constantly bouncing back and forth between negative (fixed) and positive (growth) states depending on what is at hand. As I have expressed, I like to think that we have the potential for both fixed and growth mindsets, and that these mindsets are constantly being influenced by both innate sources and our external environment. We were all born with the tools necessary to excel in at least one thing (remember in the parable of the Talents in chapter 6, every servant was given at least one Talent). However, the possibility of excelling at a plethora of things may be available to you depending on your mindset and how you face the challenges around and within you. How your life unfolds is directly dependent on the factors you welcome into your life which have the capacity to influence your mindset.

Let us first examine the external factors that you will constantly be up against when attempting to keep your mindset positive and in a growth state. Firstly, we have the **negative environment** which we discussed in the previous chapter. So, let's jump to the second and third factors: **bad habits** and **limiting beliefs**.

Bad Habits

To put it simply, bad habits are activities that you constantly engage in that add little or no true value to your life. When you engage in your bad habits you squander your time, begin procrastinating and ultimately deadlines and goals get missed. I'm sure some of you already understand or have a good sense of some of your bad habits that seem to steal your time away. If you don't, I recommend you take a few days or even a week and begin journaling, that is recording how you spend *all* your time. Audit your daily schedule for every activity you engage in including playing video games, watching TV, going out for drinks with friends etc. Analyze how your time has been spent after a week and see if there are any bad habits that you have unknowingly developed that is robbing you of time for productive, goal orientated endeavors.

I am not suggesting that you never take breaks. Of course! We have talked about exercising temperance after all. I want you to be empowered and learn how to eliminate your bad habits. *How* you spend your time will make a world of difference and set you up for a more inspiring mindset. Afterall, irrespective of our achievements, we all have 24 hours in a day. Getting closer to achieving your dreams starts with awareness and choosing to engage in more productive activities that contribute directly to your goals.

Limiting Beliefs

We grow up in a world where we are conditioned by our parents, teachers, and society to believe what they tell us. However, many of the things they teach us are invariably negative, limiting beliefs masquerading as guidance. Now, to be fair to our parents and others who we look up to (mine included), they were only sharing what had been passed on to them by their parents and teachers etc., and they believed this guidance to be true. By this our predecessor's own limiting beliefs are brought upon a new generation and further spreads. If beliefs are long standing thoughts, and your beliefs feed into your mindset which subsequently feed the mind, you can appreciate the potential impact of limiting beliefs that are brought upon you. If Columbus had believed the world was flat, he would never have made that first Journey. Have you ever paused to think of the implication of that shattered belief?

Advice offered to you throughout your life may sow the seeds of accepted limitations in your mindset which short-change your future and encourage the development of a fixed mindset. Future leaders may hold beliefs about themselves that simply are not true, or they are not willing to try to further themselves because of these held beliefs. For example, a future leader may have a held belief of, 'I am not good at Mathematics', and would never pursue any sort of study in mathematics. When you fall into this sort of habitual thought pattern of limiting yourself to what you think you are good at and bad at, it will constantly hinder your growth potential. You may come up against challenges and be willing to 'throw in the towel' as opposed to appreciating the challenge and attempting to overcome it. That is a pure fixed mindset vs a growth mindset at play.

A strong boundary to the external factors of a negative environment, bad habits and limiting beliefs is required or they will push up against your positive or growth mindset. You must be keenly aware of them and willing to continuously adjust yourself so that you can keep them from damaging your growth mindset. Let's now examine the **internal** influences that will challenge you from the inside out. One may argue that they are products of external influences, but they are marginally different. Let's examine **fear, boredom** and **stress**.

Reflection:

What bad habits can I immediately identify when examining how I spend my time?

How are these bad habits keeping me from my goals?

Are there any limiting beliefs that I keep pushing up against?

Are there any limiting beliefs that I can identify that stem from my childhood?

What sources are feeding me limiting beliefs right now that I do not need to engage with?

_____

_____

_____

_____

_____

_____

_____

Fear

This is an acronym which perfectly defines fear.

F.E.A.R.: **F**alse **E**xpectations **A**ppearing **R**eal.

Fear is crippling and stops you from moving forward. It rarely visits your mind alone and usually comes accompanied by its friend Regret: "I could've…", "I would've…" Thus, a vicious cycle is created as fear will stop you from moving forward with dreams and goals, and when you don't follow through on what your heart and mind desires, you are left with a knot of regret in your stomach. Fear is a major cause of procrastination, which is a thief of your precious time. It leads you to languish with a fixed mindset and causes you to blame everything and everyone but yourself. When you are in a fear cycle it can reveal to you that you have lost your will, are out of control and prevent further engagement with your life and aspirations.

Chemically, your fear can have a sinister effect on your brain by impairing formation of long-term memories and damaging parts of the brain such as the hippocampus (a player in your learning and memory). This can lead to diminishing the function of regulating fear which can result in you being perpetually anxious. Being in a constant state of anxiety can obviously hinder your growth mindset. If you suffer from chronic fear, you will require professional help in order to have an opportunity to live a dynamic and fruitful life. This is how damaging fear can be.

You must appreciate fear is not necessarily bad and in fact, can be very protective. When you are in actual danger of being hurt, fear will advise you how to stay safe and alive. However, you must also understand fear can be created because of internal constructs for which there is no basis. Fear is crippling and can influence your abilities and decisions. This fear may be particularly difficult to overcome, and often requires the help of professionals (such as trained therapists) to work with you through your fear slowly until you are able to overcome it.

Growing up, I had a severe case of Nyctophobia (I was afraid of the dark). I don't know what led to the germination of that fear, but it may have arisen from stories that we were told of unsavory characters lurking in the dark who are able to see you, but you are unable to see them. These stories had a great impact on me growing up and caused me to avoid dark spaces and even now as an adult, I still get a creepy feeling when I enter dark spaces. With time, I have become less fearful about entering dark spaces, but the diminution of my fear did not merely come about by me getting older. I have been led over and over into dark spaces with someone holding my hand till I was able to demonstrate that I was less fearful of the dark and can now enter dark spaces with less fear than I did previously. Occasionally though, I must confess that I still do experience hair raising anxiety on entering dark spaces.

Reflection:

How does fear show up in my life?

When was the last time I let fear stop me from moving forward with something?

Can I recall the last time I experienced a cycle of fear? How did it impact my life at the time?

_____

_____

_____

_____

_____

_____

_____

Boredom

Like fear, boredom is internally generated and it is a negative emotion you may experience daily. Now, a particular state of boredom may be beneficial when you are trying to work creatively as it can stimulate your imagination etc. However, for the sake of focusing on how you can safeguard your mindset we will just explore the type of boredom that can adversely affect your mind (even kill you). A helpful way to examine this is to understand that there are two distinct personality types that tend to suffer from boredom.

The first are people who have an impulsive personality type. They constantly need new experiences and generally find the world to be chronically under stimulating. This causes not only a sense of boredom but also anxiety and mental strain. Imagine that you have this personality type. You constantly need new experiences or to be stimulated in one way or another. Just simply going about a routine does not feel good to you. You may perceive things to be boring or find yourself reacting because things just don't seem exciting enough. This boredom is not healthy because it causes you to constantly be reactive and not being able to be in the present. You constantly look to the future as opposed to being able to remain in the present.

The second personality type finds the world at large to be a very fearful place. To remain comfortable, they will tend to shut themselves in and stay within their comfort zone, 'a type of being boxed in' at all times. Of course, these people may feel unsatisfied with life and find their day-to-day life boring. This type of boredom may be brought upon oneself. So, now imagine you are this personality type. You constantly live in fear and deny yourself from having any adventure in your life. You like to keep things under control. You aim to keep things under control so that you can remain comfortable. Of course, this brings about a sense of boredom. The unknowing moments in life can be the most exciting. So, if you are not out there living in an unknown future, then you will feel unsatisfied with your carefully curated reality.

Regardless of the personality type, these constant feelings of boredom can cause people to harm themselves. This may take the form of smoking, drinking excessive alcohol, comfort eating and experimenting with illegal drugs. It is all to alleviate boredom and try to make things more exciting or try to self soothe. On a grander scale, boredom is closely associated with depression and destructive behavior. The popular Whitehall Study done in the UK confirmed that people who were most likely to get bored were 30% more likely to die within 3 years! (This is not in line with the addition of years to your life and life to your years nor is it facilitating your growth into your excellence. For one to break the boredom cycle and thrive, you need to work on identifying the behavior, eradicate it and work on replacing it with a behavior that is more positive and productive. This is a big job especially if you have been feeling this boredom for years, but it is vital to break your relationship with boredom so that you can develop a positive mindset.

Some claim that the cycle of boredom can be easily broken by just shaking up your routine and changing the way in which you did things. The cycle can also be broken by changing your environment. Of course, knowing the reasons for the boredom may go a long way in breaking the cycle. Maybe the boredom would be the result of engaging in the habit of procrastination or you may be stuck in doing monotonous tasks. Could it be that your boredom is the result of lack of energy, direction, or focus; Maybe there is insufficient mental stimulation, you don't feel challenged enough. Whatever the cause of your boredom, it is within them you will find the clue to break the cycle.

Reflection:

Do I ever find myself bored?

What is my personality type?

Do I identify at all with being impulsive and needing stimulus all the time?

Do I feel I need to try to be in control and stay safe?

How can I combat boredom in my own life?

_____

_____

_____

_____

_____

_____

_____

_____

_____

Stress

The last internal influence on your mindset that I will discuss is stress. Stress is an enigma when it comes to its influence on your mindset. Stress can be viewed from both a fixed and growth mindset. When you are in a growth mindset stress can be seen as a welcome challenge and an opportunity to grow. On the contrary when you are in a fixed mindset, stress can lead to negative cognitive and physiological outcomes. Stress in your life may cause sleep disturbances, psychological and emotional strain leading to confusion, anxiety, and depression. In extreme cases, stress can even manifest as a psychotic illness.

The value of stress is dependent on how it is used and the impact it is allowed to have on your person. Stress is modulated by one's mindset. If you possess a growth mindset, you will see stressful situations as an opportunity to try harder. You will feel encouraged to make things happen or even to get help, thereby managing stress efficiently and effectively. Whereas if you have a fixed mindset, you are more likely to fail at managing stress. You may see stress as a sort of punishment or even as an indicator that you don't belong or can't achieve your goal. In more extreme cases, some individuals may see stress as a reason to succumb. I am sure you are familiar with or have heard of stories in which an individual simply gives up on life by committing suicide and uses the stresses they are experiencing as a motivator to end their life. Therefore, to ensure that your mind stays on the path advocated in the BMS ecosystem, of revival and vitality it is essential to manage stress in your life effectively.

Before we move on, I also want to briefly mention one of the most severe forms of stress and a newly described entity called Post Traumatic Stress Disorder (PTSD). Previously it had been thought of as an individual's construct. However, professionals have now come to understand it is an extreme reaction to a large-scale stress an individual may have experienced. There are many facets of PTSD which can include uncontrollable negative experiences or reactions which can negatively impact social relationships and one's overall quality of life. If you feel that you may be suffering from any form of PTSD, I urge you to seek professional help. There are now a variety of treatments offered that can help you get your life back.

Reflection:

Do I have a healthy relationship with stress?

Are stresses in my life affecting my health in ways such as disrupting healthy sleep cycles or causing me unwanted anxiety or depression?

When I feel stress, do I feel as if it sucks the energy out of me? Or do I feel motivated for action by the stress I feel in my life?

_____

_____

_____

_____

_____

_____

_____

_____

_____

_____

I hope you feel filled with inspiration as we complete this section of your full body revival. The mind is such an intricate and sensitive part of your being, but never forget that you have the power to stay positive and operate from a growth mindset. You will find that when you are able to do the work of reviving your mind, your life will seem brighter and more fulfilling. You will feel more energized and gain stamina to continue doing the work needed to add years to your life and life to years while growing into your excellence. When you work on your mind and its relationship to the world around you, your relationship to your precious life will also become more meaningful.

Chapter 13: Changing Mindsets

"The only constant in life is change." – Heraclitus

The Challenge

We have asserted above that both mindsets coexist in every individual, and we seem to fluctuate between one mindset and another, we also intimated that there are triggers which leads you to a change between the mindsets. The onus has also been put on you to identify those triggers. Let us look more closely at the dynamics of these mindsets and how to control or regulate them.

Since mindset is a belief system, you can begin to visualize that to change one belief system to another, the new ideas occupy the same general area in the brain as the old idea. By making the new ideas stronger, there sets up a type of competitive inhibition where the new ideas gradually become more prominent than the old idea or way of thinking, thus leading to a drift towards the thought processes engineered by the stronger ideas. The old ideas are still present, they do not disappear, but they are less dominant. Hence it is for this reason that we operate within this dynamic sea. Today or even this moment, one mindset may dominate one's thought processes, in the next moment the other mindset, whichever is stronger takes over. This mindset takeover is beckoned by the dominant belief at that time.

In medicine we learn about the placebo effect, a phenomenon in which we almost start feeling improved when a new medicine which we have been convinced should work is being used, only to find out subsequently that the medication which we believed was working was not intended to have any effect on the underlying issue. How is that possible? It is believed to be because of your belief system, a psychosomatic phenomenon. This incidentally forms the basis of cognitive therapy. By the same token we can see how some intense emotions such as anxiety, depression and anger develop. It is the result of an exaggerated interpretation of the things that we experience.

The mindset goes a bit further, it guides the interpretation process. The fixed mindset on one hand, is focused on judging. It may go along the lines of you are bad, dumb, or even superior to another. When people with a fixed mindset receive information, they tend to assimilate the information through the application of labels, that is, good information would be given a very strong positive label whilst bad information would lead to the application of a very strong negative label.

In the same vein, people with a growth mindset assimilates information they receive but the processing of that information is different, here instead of being judgmental, and self-deprecating, they are attuned towards the implication of the experience for learning and constructive action. So instead of I am bad, or I am dumb the conversation is more along the lines of what can I learn from this? How can I improve? How can I help people get better? In cognitive therapy, a very effective form of therapy, people are helped to pull back from their extreme judgements and emerge with more reasonable interpretations. Let's visit the process. Randy fails his first math test in high school, the internal conversation starts, 'You are stupid'! 'You don't belong'! In cognitive therapy Randy would be invited to analyze the information more closely by looking for evidence for and against his conclusion. A little prodding may be necessary to look at his math performance previously, this is done to identify positives that goes against his conclusion that he is stupid. Once he recognizes the positive, he becomes more amenable to trying to understand why he failed the math test. Randy is then taught how he can do this himself, so in the future when this negative self-talk visits he will be able to refute them and feel better. Earlier, I mentioned words from my father which I still revert to today as a grown man, this is refreshing and allows me to feel better and be less judgmental of myself.

Adjusting belief systems, from a fixed mindset to a growth mindset, brings about a change in perception and leaves an indelible mark on people in that it encourages a new attitude, one in which there is a willingness to make the extra effort to learn. This has the liberating consequence of allowing you to use your brain more freely and fully.

The Change

Change is easier said than done and if we must employ Heraclitus' philosophy, that change is the only constant; we would expect the change that we seek to be easy, but it needs direction and encouragement, guidance if you will.

One must understand that in attempting to move from a fixed mindset to a growth mindset, people hold on to the fixed mindset for a reason. It must have proven useful to them at some point in their life. It told them how their parents and teachers perceived them, and they accepted it because it led to the development of a type of behavior which allowed the children to feel loved and protected, on the contrary, as a child purposeful deviation from that position would cause children to feel loss, unloved and alone. The equation here is not balanced and children we know need to feel supported and loved. With that seed sewn, the children had to find a way to feel safe, loved and to win their parents and seniors over, so they unquestionably believed what they were told. In that moment the purpose of a fixed mindset is not only given birth too, but it serves a useful purpose, that of acceptance, protection, and love. These children therefore grow into this mindset and so will be resistant to change, their very behavior will be conditioned on the validation of that mindset, the fixed mindset.

In trying to effect change in people's mindset, we are asking people to give up the mindset which has served them well over the years, giving them an identity and self-esteem. It is even more difficult where the converse of this, the new concept that you must adhere to, advises the embrace of all things that threatens the posture of a fixed mindset. You are now being schooled to accept and embrace challenges, struggle, criticism and setbacks and to accept effort on your part to gain access to this new dispensation.

It must also be understood that the fixed mindset till then is comfortable and is not willing to give up its position. It will therefore cause you to feel less good about yourself. You may feel that your value as a person is deteriorating. Remember the fixed mindset previously offered you security for which you may still yearn, so it willing offers it up again. You may feel that you descend into the sea of sameness, just ordinary drifting away from the pedestal you once occupied. It may initially prove difficult to grasp, but opening yourself up to growth makes you more yourself, giving you the option to become who you really are. There is a truth about the process.

Developing the Growth Mindset

We have all applied for positions in our lives that we were unable to secure for whatever reason, the first time around. Our reaction to that rejection will serve as a template of what happens next.

We always have options; in this case do we react to this rejection with a fixed mindset frame or with that of a growth mindset.

With the fixed mindset frame, we see the rejection as a challenge to our self-esteem and so we may start making excuses or being judgmental with the situation, conversely, with some self-talk you start rationalizing the reason for your non-acceptance. Since in a growth mindset you are determined to use each setback as a learning experience, you set out to determine why your application was rejected. You call the responsible party who reviews your application, he likes your initiative, and invites you for an interview which you can scale and get offered the job. Embracing rejection as an opportunity for learning, a key feature of the growth mindset. This is but a single step in the mindset development. Once you get offered the job, the learning should continue for the continued development of this mindset which appears to be proactive.

Having specific, vivid, concrete plans also helps. Being able to make your plans so vivid that you can virtually see it unfold is a great stimulus to allowing the plan to be birthed. The idea is not simply to make a growth mindset plan but to have a precise, vivid, concrete plan about

145

the execution. You must not only visualize the plan, but you must stick to it.

Entitlement: The Problem

Does the world owe us? With a fixed mindset our belief system may drift in the direction that the world owes us. How many times do we allow our thought to drift into thinking that people should see your talents and reward you. When this does not happen, your conclusion is that it is not fair. You just want what you consider is yours. For a longtime you thought of yourself as superior, but you have now begun to realize that you are an ordinary, run-of-the-mill individual, which is not what you want to be. You are not feeling good about yourself because you seem to be in the same category of people you despise and feel superior too. It then dawns on you that some people stand out because of their effort and commitment. You start putting more effort in and pay attention to the rewards that result. It may take some time before you begin to enjoy putting in the effort as well as learning.

Many people with a fixed mindset eventually understand that their cloak of specialness was a mere façade they developed much like a cocoon to allow them to feel safe, strong, and worthy. While it offered protection early on, it morphed with time into a constricting feature limiting their growth and sending them into self-defeating battles which effectively cuts them off from satisfying mutual relationships.

The Process

Change though constant, is not easy. Changing mindsets is not easy, though we recognize that going from a fixed mindset to a growth mindset is the commendable path. It is a process which requires nourishment, ongoing support, and maintenance. There are several steps involved in the conversion from a fixed mindset to a growth mindset. Afterall, the fixed mindset played a role up to now in your growth, so it may be uncomfortable to shed what you know for what you do not know, and the fixed mindset is comfortable in its home and will not willing give way to a new construct. It will remain but needs to coexist with this new mindset and therefore will be in constant competition with it. To adopt a predominant growth mindset, the equation must be weighted in the direction of the growth mindset.

$$\text{Fixed Mindset} \quad \rightleftharpoons \quad \text{Growth mindset}$$

I believe that for a change to be realized there must be an increased influence by the growth mindset, a feature which can only be developed by extending support and nourishment to the growth mindset. This is, however, a process involving several steps.

- Step 1: would be an embrace of the fixed mindset. Understand its presence and be prepared to work with it.

- Step 2: would be to understand and be familiar with its triggers. What triggers its appearance? Is it stress? Is it the breaking of new ground? Is it the unknown? You need to identify its triggers and its behavior.

- Step 3: Be familiar with its behavior and so identify its personality. Name that personality, my preference would be to give it a name that you don't like.

- Step 4: When that personality shows up talk to it, listen to its urgings and discuss why you are embarking on this journey. Invite him to join you on the journey.

With this approach, you will morph from the fixed mind set towards your preferred growth mindset and it will also ensure your continued nourishing of your preferred mindset.

We have covered reviving your body and mind. It is now time to dive into the beauty of your spirit and how it relates to your life and the world around you. You have some exciting and important work ahead!

PART 3: THE SPIRIT

"There are no constraints on the human mind, no walls around the human spirit, no barriers to our progress except those we ourselves erect." – Ronald Reagan

Humankind is a complex entity composed of a physical body, a mind, and a spirit. These components work synergistically, to create a fully functional being. The interrelationship suggests that each component can impact the other component. As you may recall we refer to this as a triune, where three different entities co-exist to comprise a whole. We have examined your body which is readily understood as we can explore it through our five senses. We have also examined your mind, which you cannot see or touch, but you can observe it at work through the outcomes, behavior, and personalities. It is now time to examine and discuss your spirit. It is the other component which makes up your person.

However, it takes a bit more open-mindedness as the Spirit is not readily observed, though our emotions are a fair indication of the status of our spirit. The presence of our spirit continues to influence your day-to-day activities.

Chapter 14: The Human Spirit

"I believe very deeply in the human spirit, and I have a sense of awe about it. I look around and ask, what makes the difference? What is it? I have known people the world has thrown everything at – to discourage them, to kill them, to break their spirit! And yet something about them retains a dignity. . ." – Horton Foote

The Spirit

There are countless terminologies used to refer to the human spirit, as well as explanations of its functions and the rationale for its existence. Permit me the opportunity to analyze a few commonly held views here.

Scholars have noted that there is a physical and non-physical world coexisting. The spirit is thought to be part of the non-physical world, a vibrational energy that we cannot see, cannot create, nor destroy. Some people believe that our spirit marshals our intellect, emotions, fears, passions, and creativity.

There is no denying that our spirit is a part of us and may have either a healthy or unhealthy relationship with our mindset and body. Defining the spirit will help you to understand and allow for a development and interaction that fosters stretching of yourself as you grow into your excellence.

Some define the spirit in terms of energy, sticking to the natural law that energy cannot be created nor destroyed. The view that the spirit cannot be created nor destroyed is universal and as such is without argument. Some may argue that it fails to address the origin of energy. Some proponents of that view revert to the bible for an explanation and claim that by the creator breathing into the nostrils of man at the time of his creation to enliven him was tantamount to the passage of the spirit to man. Even today, life of man begins with the inhalation of the first breath whereas life ends with the exhalation of his last breath. It is believed that the breath returns to the creator. Breath then is described by the proponents of that belief as the spirit, the energy. There may be scriptural support for this belief in Genesis chapter 2 verse 7. ....and breathed into his nostrils the breath of life; and man became a living soul. In Ecclesiastes chapter 12 verse 7; it states then shall the dust return to the earth as it was: and the spirit shall return unto God who gave it. It will be noted in the story of creation, the breath is the only item which was passed directly from the creator to mankind. Yet the lower animals also have breath, although there is no documented biblical evidence that this breath was passed directly from the creator to animals. Some contend that animals have spirits, but the biblical evidence is lacking.

Secondly, Christians talk of the holy spirit. One is now left to wonder whether there is a difference between the spirit of man and the holy spirit. Remember, if the spirit of man is the same as the holy spirit, there would be a biblical argument in support of this assumption, additionally some may argue that there may be evidence that they are not the same. Let's explore what is known. The creator as taught by the Christian faith is composed of three entities in one, the Father, the son, and the holy spirit. During creation, the creator blew into the nostrils of man to begin life and at the end of his sojourn on earth the breath returns to the creator. If the creator is composed of three entities, one of which is the holy spirit, it seems logical to accept the teaching of Christianity that the holy spirit is what was blown into man to start life. Arguably though, the lower animals also breathe to start life, so are we assuming that these lower animals also possess the holy spirit? Surely not, the bible tells us that the creator made man in his own image which upon reflection is composed of a father, the son, and a holy spirit; animals were not made in the creator's image. This would seem to put to rest the notion that the breath is the spirit but if it is, why was mankind's received by special delivery? Directly from the creator! Additionally, the bible is filled with evidence which clearly indicates that the breath is not the holy spirit. If nothing else, Christianity's claim that the holy spirit was sent after man's creation and was to be a comforter, clearly is bible evidenced based. The question becomes, why duplication? Inherently though the human spirit and the holy spirit are not the same. The bible also speaks about the fruits of the spirit and talks about evil spirits, allowing us to distinguish one from the other. The fruits of the spirit are defined as: Love, Joy, Peace, Patience, Kindness, Goodness, Gentleness, Faithfulness, and Self-control. If this spirit exists in mankind, what will lend support to Jeremy's apparent evidenced based conviction?

Others like Jeremy Griffith in his book, 'Freedom the end of the human condition describes the human condition as a paradox, he claims: The human condition is our species extraordinary capacity for what has been called 'good' and 'evil.' He goes on to say, while it is undeniable that human beings are capable of great love and empathy, we also have an unspeakable history of greed, hatred, rape, torture, murder, and war; a propensity for deeds so shocking and overwhelming that the eternal question of why, seems depressingly inexplicable. Even in our everyday behavior, when the ideals of life are to be cooperative, selfless, and loving are we so ruthlessly competitive, selfish, and aggressive that human life has become all but unbearable and our planet near destroyed. Surely, that description of the human condition seems far removed from the holy spirit and its fruits.

Rhonda Byrne, the author of 'The Secrets', seems to avoid contradiction and prefers to refer to the human spirit as simply the universe. This she seemingly credits with a phenomenon referred to as the law of attraction.

I have always felt that there is an incompleteness with man's behavior, through-out his history, he seems to crave for something beyond him; a being or object outside of himself to pay homage too and worship. To avoid this discussion from degenerating into a religious discussion or a Christianity versus a non-Christian approach, or a bible believer versus a non-believer. The rest of the discussion of the spirit will be through the eyes of the amalgamation of these views to avoid alienating any belief system.

Emotion

The Spirit is like an emotion, that is, we know it exists but cannot touch it and may not be able to rationalize its existence. This is distinct from the mindset, although it may be able to influence our mindset and thought process. Allow me to clarify. Fear, for example, is an emotion which can be brought on by what our thoughts tell us, for example, If we think we are going to be attacked by a dog that will generate the emotion of fear, but is that mindset? Surely not? Is that simply a thought, of course it is but it produces an emotion.

The neuroscientist tells us that there is both a subjective and objective assessment of thought. Subjectively, the neuroscientist claims that our thoughts come from nowhere; they just pop into our heads or emerge in the form of words leaving our mouths. Objectively, our thoughts emerge from neural processes which come from everywhere. Whereas in the previous section, we learnt that our mindset is a product of our thoughts which we have held unto and as a result, this developed into a belief system which leads to our mindset that directs our activities; we recognize that some of our thoughts have an emotional component, and it is this component of our thoughts that feeds our spirit.

As we go through this section, we will learn about the existence of the emotional guidance system (EGS) which indicates the appropriateness of what is fed to our spirit. We learnt in section 2 that our mindset is nourished by our thoughts, the chronicity of which generates our belief system. We are now being introduced to the way our thoughts influence our spirit through the generation of emotions. If our thoughts are appropriate, we will tend to have our emotions moving in the direction of level 1 on the EGS.

We can therefore begin to sense the interconnectedness of the components of the triune. Our bodies, mind, and spirit act harmoniously to produce the final product, who we manifest.

The Role of Your Spirit

You may identify your Spirit as that small voice inside you that helps you to decipher right from wrong. It is that entity one occasionally describes as your conscience, your morals which guides you along the path considered right by you based on your training and exposure. Your spirit may comfort you in times of need and your very spirit may even act as an advocate. In the bible it is said that we are made in God's image, and God is a spirit, so it is palpably obvious then that we too have a spiritual component. But what exactly is the spirit? We cannot touch, feel, see, smell, or taste it. Is it a figment of our imagination? Surely, we can recognize the workings of the spirit which can be manifested through our emotions, and it yields or bears results or fruits. We have referred to people from time to time as having a cheerful spirit, a kind spirit, a forgiving spirit etc. Giving credence to the view that our spirit can be reflected in our emotions.

Many believe that our spirit is linked to an authority greater than us and is our vehicle which allows us to connect with the greater good allowing the receipt of gifts and power into our lives. The Bible says if we ask for anything, it shall be given. The teachings of Abraham-Hicks are based on the understanding that the non-physical world has an abundance to offer you, but you must ask for it. Rhonda Bryne, the author of "The Secret" approaches it from a similar but slightly different angle when she proposes we can gain whatever we ask of the universe through one of the natural laws, The Law of Attraction. Mastin Kipp (leadership coach) teaches that the number one hindrance people have working against them is that they do not believe success is possible for them. As you can see, all these ideas from great thought leaders and scripture have in common, a belief. Believing first that there is something more than just the life you can see and feel. Being willing to ask for what you want and finally believing that you shall receive it, through some apparent magic, facilitates the delivery and your receipt of that for which you asked. The adage that anything the mind of man can perceive (think of) and believe that it can achieve. If looked at differently, we understand that we must first have a dream, but that is not enough. We must believe that the dream is possible (the belief is essential). It is an emotion, hence nourishment for the spirit, and because we know it is possible, our belief system takes over, our spirit is appropriately nourished, and our spirit facilitates the rendering of our request. This is virtually identical to faith which is commonly referred to among those of a Christian persuasion.

Faith

Faith in religious circles is defined as the substance of things hoped for, the evidence of things not seen. The literature on hope is equivocal, it says that hope is at least not a fundamental emotion because hope is situation specific and contingent on one's own abilities. Yet hoping for an item is not contingent on our own abilities and in that context therefore, hope is an emotion. By extrapolation, then, if we accept hope as an emotion, and we define faith as the substance of an emotion, faith must therefore be an emotion and hence potential nourishment for our spirit. This is almost identical to bible verse (Mark11:24) that says whatever you ask for in prayer, believe that you have received it, and it will be yours. To receive it, you must have faith, you must display the emotion of belief, the spirit must be appropriately nourished. The spirit world has a limitless supply of goodies for us to tap into, our spiritual component allows us to tap into these boundless goodies but to obtain them we must ask, believe, and exercise faith, that is nourish our spirit appropriately. Both belief and faith are emotions and are therefore potential nourishment for our spirit. If our belief and faith are aligned, then the appropriate nourishment of our spirit will result, we will then move forwards on the emotional guidance system (EGS).

This is quite similar, almost identical to Abraham-Hicks's teachings but expressed very differently. Abraham-Hicks prefers to view the interaction in terms of vibrations. He implies that if our vibrations or emotions are aligned, we will move forwards along the EGS.

Rhonda Bryne, the author of the secret, addresses the same subject and speaks of the natural Law, the Law of attraction. This law as stated claims that like attract like. Unfortunately, this law does not withstand scrutiny in the manner stated.

Since our belief system originates from our thoughts and the emotional component of our thoughts nourishes our spirit, your spirit revolves around your own belief system. You must ask yourself if you are willing to believe there is more to your life than just what you can see or feel whether stepping out of your own way, out of your comfort zone to achieve, is a necessary step to facilitate your growth into your excellence. We are aware that we are promised anything we ask of the universe. It simply says ask and you shall receive, we are further chided almost mockingly, when we are told the reason we don't have is because we don't ask. We are left with no excuse but to ask, in asking however we must have faith or believe that our request shall be granted. The popular teaching that what you believe you can achieve is not far-fetched, but you must be willing to receive and to that I add, you must be prepared to give thanks. For by showing appreciation for your gifts, you encourage the universe to give more. Remember the story of the parable in chapter 6.

The Christian teachings is that when you ask, you get one of three responses: **YES, NO** or **NOT YET** (though there is no biblical support for the **NO** response). All the bible specifically states is, ask, and it shall be given! Others interpret the offer differently, claiming that there is a three-step process involved. The interpretations are almost identical but the response from a request is never no. It is always given as per the statement in the bible; ask and it shall be given. According to the teachings of Rhonda Byrne and other proponents of the Law of attraction, there is need for alignment of vibrations, with that said, If the alignment of vibrations is not harmonious, the request made is not granted, some would interpret this as a 'no' response.

The interpretation of the Christians **'not yet'** response is based on your level of preparedness for the receipt of the requested item. A similar explanation is advanced by those who believe in making a request to the universe, if there appears to be a delay in your receipt of the requested item, the individuals leaning to request items from the universe, will interpret this delay as either a **'no'** response or a **'not yet'** response. They then seek to justify their claim by indicating that the universe did not believe/think or feel that you were sufficiently prepared to receive the item which you requested, hence the response, **'NO'**. This explanation gives life to the universe, so is this a succinct hint of the existence of a greater being? Unfortunately, I disagree with the Christian teaching here, as there is no biblical support for a 'NO' response. The bible does say that God will repay each according to his deed. Is that the context in which the apparent 'NO' should be interpreted? The 'not yet' response, though those of a Christian persuasion may interpret this to be the result of a lack of faith! We must recall that there was no time given when your goodies which you requested from the universe would be made available to you. We were simply advised that if we asked, it would be given. Is the delay in receiving our requested goodies the result of a lack of faith?

The Christian teachings seem to suggest that the greater your faith, the more likely you will receive the request which you have made, a sort of **quid pro quo** arrangement. The biblical evidence for this seems to be lacking.

In none of the biblical texts quoted does it give an indication that a request is never answered or put on hold. Advice has always been to ask, and it shall be given unto you. To obtain clarity, I tried to question the use of shall in that statement as opposed to will. Both words talk of future events but there are two basic English rules which govern their use. Additionally, there is a difference between a strong and a normal future event. Grammatically correct English uses 'shall' to address normal future events when using the first person such as I and/or We. Will is used to reflect normal future events in the second and third person (you, it, or they). In strong future events, there is more of an emotional component to the future and the roles of will and shall are reversed, with this in mind let us review the statement, ask and it (third person) shall be given unto you. Inherent in that statement is the strong future that it (third person)

159

shall be given unto you. Since our spirit is nourished by our emotions, was it a deliberate play on words to ensure our spirit is appropriately nourished in the process? Remember the emotional component of our thoughts nourishes our spirit. Note the roles are reversed so to relay the strength of the future and ensuring its emotional content, the word shall is used. It is a promise laced with emotions. Interestingly, the term does not give a finite time during which your request will be granted. What we do know, however, is that it shall be granted. So, from the biblical promise all we can claim is that our request shall be granted but we do not know when, herein may lie the basis of the **'Not Yet'** response, hence the need for both faith and patience.

Visualization and Faith

Faith is defined as the substance of things hoped for, the evidence of things not seen. A new entity is brought forth, 'hope without seeing that which you requested'. Inherent in the definition of hope is there a silent implication that in the process of acquiring that which you ask for, you must be prepared to paint as clear a picture of what you can, as if you are able to see what you requested. In other words, we are asked to move beyond the physical. Hope is defined as a feeling of expectation and desire for a particular event to occur. Taking this definition and relating it to the Christian teaching of a need for more faith would complicate interpretation by suggesting that there are degrees of feelings of expectation. Naturally our expectations in everyday life waver, so is this what is required to be brought under control to ensure we achieve that which we requested if we are to avoid the **'NOT YET'** response? Other interpretations of the workings of the spirit traverse similar paths without establishing a bridge, an entity which appears to be painfully necessarily obvious in elucidating the issue.

The concept of faith hints at emotion without stating so but let us look more closely at the accepted meaning of faith and analyze what is being said. We claim that faith is the substance of things hoped for, the evidence of things not seen. We will quickly realize that hope generates an expectation, an emotion if you will, in us. Hope is fundamentally not an emotion, and it is very situation specific. It may be contingent on our own abilities. The second part of the definition of Faith.... the evidence of things not seen... instils within us clarity that our emotions are brought into play. Why the specific reference on the visual. Does that suggest the need to paint as clear a picture as possible of what you hope to achieve? It also injects the need for a belief. Combined we have a hope (a situation specific entity capable of generating an emotion and we have evidence, though we cannot see it, but it generates belief) and belief. We have a believable emotion that is tantamount to faith. Obviously, therefore, we ask (ask and it shall be given unto you) and we have the belief that we will receive, through faith, must be precisely visualized imaginatively, (the believable emotion). Our emotions will reflect happiness which will take us forwards on the EGS. This will automatically start paying us a dividend, as the happiest, most positive people tend to be the healthiest, most successful, most generous, and even the most popular. Hence are better primed to grow into excellence. Positivity is contagious. This positivity therefore feeds back into your mindset and benefits not only you but everyone around you. Interestingly, a positive emotion is thought to generate a stronger response than a negative one.

Above we mentioned that our spirit is both an advocate and a comforter, both tasks we can readily observe are designed to make you happy. We can now appreciate the role of positive psychology, the scientific study of positive human emotion, happiness, and well-being. Emanating from this realm of science is the realization that positivity can benefit all aspects of human life and health. There is therefore an inevitable need for the contribution from the spirit if we are to benefit from the addition of years to our lives and life to our years while growing into our excellence.

Abraham-Hicks's teachings have a different take on how things are acquired. As per his teachings, the source of all goodies is the universe which has an inexhaustible supply. To obtain anything from this abundance, you only need to request it. Abraham-Hicks contends, though he does not reference it, that all you need to do is to make the request. He also indicates that there is a three-step process before one can accept his requested goodies:

1. The request (which, as per Abraham-Hicks and the bible is always granted)

2. The Granting of the request

3. The receipt of the goodies.

It is at #3 that Abraham-Hicks teachings deviate from the biblical teachings. Though the bible does not give an explanation, it is obvious that if something is given it must be received. The bible does not detail the receiving process, it leaves a void which may be filled by differing interpretations. Nature abhors a vacuum. Abraham-Hicks seems to suggest that the void may be bridged, if you follow his insight on vibrational energy, according to your vibrations and the vibrations of your request. These vibrations, I venture to say are directed by the magnetizer, our focus.

The belief is if your vibrations and the vibrations of your request are in alignment, you will receive that which you requested. The contention that a shift in your vibrations will lead you to emotional evidence, that is if your vibrations and the vibrations of your request are in alignment you will experience a shift in your emotional guidance system towards the pole of happiness, but it won't yield instant physical evidence of the goodies you requested. The obvious question is, is this not the definition of faith? The evidence of things not seen!! From that standpoint it appears that Abraham-Hick's interpretation of the process is closer to the bible's teachings than the interpretation of the Christian leadership. It also explains the delay and possibly failure to receive the requested goodies.

Rhonda Bryne, the author of "The Secret" approaches it from a similar but slightly different angle when she proposes we can gain whatever we ask of the universe through the activity of a natural law, the law of attraction. This law implies an operative mechanism described as vibrations and suggests numerous strategies that produce appropriate vibrations which move your emotional state in a positive direction. Among some of the suggested approaches is the gratitude stacking method. Here the advice is to make a list of anything for which you are grateful, be it material objects, an event, or some pleasant memory. The number of items on your list depends on you. There is also the time-lapse method in which a list is made of anything that you have had, anything that you have or anything you wish to have. In this case the list should be comprised of about 15 items, in no specific pattern, items had, items have, and items hoped for all jumbled in no particular sequence and you give thanks for each item. The rationale given for the effectiveness of this method is based on the realization that 66% of your listed items have already manifested, it seeks to explain that on going through that list there is a certainty in your vibration that carries over and applies to the future items (those hoped for). It is felt that it is easier and more natural for your body to regulate your emotions by not allowing it to stray too far from the items on the list. Superficially, this makes sense but does this principle obtain? The proponents believe that it works.

Mastin Kipp believes that the number-one hindrance to success is people who believe it is not possible for them. He says if you believe something is not possible then you are right. And the whole universe will conspire to prove you are right, not because the universe is a bad place but because that is how you are interacting with it, and you'll find yourself looking for proof to support your belief, why it is not possible.

In essence, in attempting to bridge this void all the authors quoted are basically saying the same thing which we will have a closer look at in this section.

The workings of the spirit within you allow some great emotional characteristics to emerge which are referred to as the fruits of the spirit, all seemingly good qualities which coat you with a veneer that we should all aspire to. The fruits are love, joy, peace, forbearance, kindness, goodness, faithfulness, gentleness, and self-control. All traits, I am sure you will agree, help us to be better versions of ourselves and facilitate better interpersonal relationships thus encouraging your growth into your excellence.

If your spirit is shining forth within you, a bystander would be expected to recognize the unavoidable love that you show for your fellow man, your happiness will be clearly and readily be identifiable and you would obviously be at peace with your environment, neighbors, and colleagues. The fruits of forbearance, kindness, goodness, and faithfulness are all virtues we love to see in our fellow men and with gentleness and self-control thrown in, a collection of emotions that we can display and are manifested by us in varying degrees but together makes our neighbors and associates comfortable with us. Aspiring to the acquisition of these virtues is commendable and will doubtlessly facilitate the growth into your excellence.

Reflection:

How do I identify my spirit?

When have I felt my spirit evident in my life?

When was the last time I exhibited faith in my life?

Do I show appreciation and gratitude for my gifts?

Make a list of the last five gifts for which you have been grateful.

Should I be doing things differently to really prove that I am grateful?

How may I nurture the "fruits" of the spirit in my life? (love, joy, kindness, etc.)

_____

_____

_____

_____

_____

_____

_____

_____

_____

_____

In the following chapters of this section, I will explore how you nourish, that is cultivate and maintain these attributes, I will also explore the optimum environment in which these traits flourish and finally I will explore factors which we allow to affect our spirits.

Chapter 15: Nourishing Your Spirit

"There's nothing more nourishing to the spirit than doing what you feel called to do." – Megan Shull

Feeding the Spirit

Any living object which is nourished reflects the appropriateness of that nourishment through changes, usually growth of some kind. The spirit is no exception. To appreciate the effectiveness of the nourishment provided to your spirit we will need to discuss the emotional guidance system (EGS). Briefly we have learnt that when our bodies are appropriately nourished, we have a change in our physical bodies and their function. The effect of both over and under nourishment of our bodies is readily visible in our environment. Similarly, the appropriateness of the nourishment of our mindset impacts the way we think and behave. We see the effect of this among the dreamers and their accomplishments in our environment. Nourishment of our spirit leads to a change in our emotional states, be it leading to happiness or its inverse, sadness. Though we may not yet appreciate how this change in emotional states came by, we have doubtlessly seen it in action among our peers and those who cross our paths. I believe that to gain a clear understanding of how nourishment of our spirit impacts our emotional state we must visit the EGS on which we will clarify how nourishment of any type positive or negative impacts our spirit by leading to changes in our emotional states.

Your spirit is waiting to offer you a bounty of goodness. Caring for your spirit is essential when looking to elevate your life. If you nourish your spirit appropriately it will reward you, no doubt! This is part of its design.

What is nourishment for your spirit, and how can it be best provided?

Nourishing your spirit involves taking care of your emotions. As mentioned before the emotional component of your thoughts is the nourishment for your spirit and in turn helps your spirit to be free to give back to you. Like a Global Positioning System (GPS) that you may use when driving or travelling, which gives you the guidance to get to your desired destination, you have an internal navigation system that you are born with which helps guide you through various emotional states to the preferred emotional state of your spirit. It is referred to as your Emotional Guidance System (EGS) which is inherently a part of you and reflects the status of your spirit. You can think of your EGS as a co-pilot in your emotional life. Just as a GPS system navigates you towards your destination from point A to B, your emotions move you along your EGS towards one or the other pole on the EGS. Pleasant emotions which reflect the fruits of the spirit will move you towards happiness, whilst the reverse is true.

The Emotional Guidance System (EGS)

The Emotional Guidance System is composed of a variety of levels of emotions which are listed from number 1 to 21. The various emotional levels which comprise the EGS are listed below. Your spirit is more appropriately nourished as your emotions move closer towards level 1. (The spirit prefers that you remain on the emotional trajectory going towards level # 1.). This is necessary to allow the universe to deliver the goodies you requested.

1. Joy/Knowledge/Empowerment/ Freedom/Love/Appreciation

2. Passion

3. Enthusiasm/Eagerness/Happiness

4. Positive Expectation/Belief

5. Optimism

6. Helpfulness

7. Contentment

8. Boredom

9. Pessimism

10. Frustration/Irritation/Impatience

11. Overwhelm

12. Disappointment

13. Doubt

14. Worry

15. Blame

16. Discouragement

17. Anger/Revenge

18. Hatred/Rage

19. Jealousy

20. Insecurity/Guilt/Unworthiness

21. Fear/Grief/Depression/Despair/Powerlessness/Stress

Note that as you get closer to the top of the list you encounter happier emotions. As you go down the list the emotions continue to become less desirable. You want to try to steer away from the less desirable emotions. When nourishing your spirit, you can track the appropriateness of the nourishment with your EGS. The more appropriate the nourishment, the better your emotional state as the movement up your EGS heads towards level one. You can track in which direction you are going, because as you move in the direction of level one, you feel happier and have a greater sense of joy because you are moving towards your ideal emotional state to welcome great things into your life and the growth into your excellence. What creates this movement from one emotion to the next is your thoughts. Not only do your thoughts establish your belief system and feed your mindset; but your thoughts are massaged by your spirit. Your spirit has an inseparable relationship with your mindset. Your emotions direct the emotional guidance system and determine the direction of migration along the emotional guidance system. Your thoughts in turn are guided by your position on the EGS. Your thoughts determine your behavior, and your thoughts eventually develop into your mindset. In the teachings of Abraham-Hicks these thoughts are manifested as a vibrational energy which feeds the spirit and brings it into alignment with your desire. The energy created by this vibration helps move you along this emotional guidance system towards your desired goal.

You must be prepared to show gratitude for your gifts. Through your expression of gratitude, you encourage your spirit to give more and more. When you are willing to remain open to the possibility that there is more to you than just your body and your mind, your spirit will work synergistically with these two components to create a state of balance and harmony and provide you with your request. When you can find this balance, you will truly set yourself up for a complete revival of self, adding years to your life and life to your years as well as aid in the growth into your excellence.

It brings us back to the idea of what you can conceive and believe, you can achieve. Your EGS will be the perfect guide to your emotional state and indicate the suitability of the nourishment to your spirit. The more adequately your spirit is nourished by positivity and encouraging emotional plaudits, essentially operant conditioning, the closer you will be to the higher levels of the EGS and, in return, more in line with achieving your goals. The use of planful operations and operant conditioning methods, such as positive self-appraisal, the smoother is your transition along the emotional positioning system, and the more nourishing it is to the spirit. Appreciation through the expression of gratitude for your gifts also helps to nourish the spirit. The way you choose to show appreciation is immaterial. Some degree of satisfaction is always evoked by saying thanks. It is also believed by some that the process involved in showing gratitude alters and redirects your vibrations. This facilitates nourishment of your spirit and leads to the movement in the direction of the happier pole of the emotional guidance system. Let's look at an example of how the EGS works in your life.

Let us suppose you wanted to make more money. As we now know, the Universe is filled with abundance, and you must be willing to receive that for which you asked. But what if you are faced with a belief that there are no more jobs available that will pay more than you currently earn? This brings you into a particular vibrational state that is not in line with receiving more money into your life. There is no belief more money is available to you, your vibration therefore, will not be appropriately aligned and you are blocking the receipt of more money. You are not prepared to receive that for which you ask, so your vibrations would not be in sync, and you would drop to a lower level on the EGS. In examining your emotional state, you are in DOUBT, #13 on the EGS. Now, what if you moved your emotional state into DISAPPOINTMENT, because you realize that you haven't really put in the effort to investigate all possibilities for finding new work. It may still feel negative, but in fact it has brought you up to #12 on the EGS. You have improved your vibrational state, through the nourishment of your spirit. #11 OVERWHELM may then come into play by putting some effort into looking for a new job. All these small tweaks in your emotions will continue to effectively nourish your spirit and move you into a more compatible vibration guiding you in the appropriate direction up your EGS. Your emotions will improve, and your spirit will be more nourished. Keeping in mind the adage, "by the yard it's hard, by the inch it's a cinch!" can really help you appreciate the relationship between your spirit, your emotions, and your mindset. Rarely will you find that you suddenly skip a bunch of emotions and find yourself at an elevated level along the EGS. It is usually small but meaningful steps in the direction which brings you the greatest joy.

Let us pause to temporarily look at those two emotional states, **(a) DOUBT** and (b) **DISAPPOINTMENT**.

Doubt and Disappointment

Doubt you will realize has a crippling effect on your emotions, there is a lack of belief and hence a lack of drive because you do not believe that there is better. There is no alignment with the vibrations. You are asking the universe for a particular gift, but you doubt you will receive it, hence leading to a lack of synchronicity in emotional vibrations. You then succumb to your doubts and hence belief that there is nothing better or that it is not achievable. Does that seem to create a platform on which excuses are built? On closer assessment, this is almost identical to the thought process of a person with a fixed mindset. Could it be that the ego is at work here, offering protection against embarrassment. (S)he doubts that there is anything better so (s)he remains in his/her comfort zone. If we look at the emotions 13 to 21 on the EGS, they seem to be more commonly found in people with a fixed mind set.

The emotion of disappointment reflects the emotional state of someone who has begun the process of reflection. (S) He has started to become a participant in his/her own existence. There is an attempt to question what has been happening to you and as you reflect the emotion of disappointment sweeps over you as you begin to realize more could have been done. This quasi-self-assessment extends to level 8 on the EGS, the emotional state of boredom. The various emotional states from level

12 to level 8 reflect a vibration of a mindset in transition between a fixed mindset and a growth mindset. The other levels up to level 1 are more commonly associated with a growth mindset. Again, reflecting the interconnectedness between the mindset and the spirit, these two together will encourage the physical structure of your body to act. This provides further evidence that all three compartments of the triune clearly work synergistically to project the person you are.

This is where having faith can be of comfort. Appropriate nourishment to your spirit will undoubtedly help you climb higher in your EGS. However, you must start from a place of belief. If we define faith as the substance of things hoped for, the evidence of things not seen, we can more clearly see how faith fits into the functioning of the EGS.

Faith helps because there may be no physical evidence of your desires for a long time. You must stay strong and on top of remembering that "if you believe it, you can achieve it" you must also bring yourself into a state of *feeling* like you already are living or experiencing that for which you ask.... This will doubtlessly provide nourishment for the spirit. If we refer to the previous example, you must feel like you are already making more money before you see evidence of it. This is such an important final piece to nourish the spirit. This is analogous to Hicks's third component in the process of obtaining gifts from the universe. It may really stretch you mentally especially if you are new to the concept of nourishing the spirit (an integral aspect to understanding the BMS ecosystem.) But you must have faith, and trust (believe) that your efforts in raising your vibrational energy will not fail.

Reflection:

If I think of something that is happening right now in my life or a goal that I am consciously working on, can I pinpoint where I am on my EGS?

In this instance, how can I move up the EGS?

Are there a few examples that I can flush out for myself?

Can I reflect on moments in my life where I have felt each emotion on the EGS?

Can I relate each emotion to the one above and understand how my vibrations can take me to a higher emotional state?

_____

_____

_____

_____

_____

_____

_____

_____

_____

_____

_____

_____

I hope you are feeling as excited as I was when I first learned about my EGS. It is an eye opening and inspiring way of ensuring appropriate alignment with the components of the self. While it may take some internal adjusting, learning how your emotions and vibrational states interact. It is essential to the growth process as you grow into your excellence within the BMS ecosystem.

Levels 1 to 7 (Happiness Zone) at the top of the EGS, are the emotions of Joy, Knowledge, Empowerment, Freedom, Love, Appreciation; Passion, Enthusiasm, Eagerness and Happiness compare this with the stated fruits of the spirit; Love, Joy, Peace, Patience, Kindness, goodness, faithfulness, gentleness, and self-control. These Levels seem in capsule form to be an embodiment of the fruits of the spirit. Let us look more closely at one such emotion, **happiness**.

Happiness

Most experts on the science of happiness agree that the term does not refer to fleeting sensations of joy or pleasure. Being happy does not mean that you feel great all the time, nor does it mean that you're always in a good mood. Research suggests that people who experience the greatest overall well-being are not specifically susceptible to intense emotional highs, this is preferred, because such emotional highs are usually accompanied by intense lows. Life on an emotional plateau is more rewarding than life on an emotional roller coaster. Life on an emotional roller coaster would be akin to one diagnosed with bipolar disorder. Further, it must be noted that feeling good all the time is not attainable.

Science is clear that happiness is not about material possessions. Happiness is related to having a sense of overall satisfaction with life. It is a sense of fulfilment combined with an overall feeling of well-being that you experience daily. This does not mean that a happy person will not have to deal with sadness, anger, or despair, but they know that these feelings are fleeting, they did not come to stay and yes, they will pass. You need to learn how to tolerate and overcome them.

Relationship Breakdown

Those who succeed and excel in their area of expertise are found to be the individuals who are most happy with their chosen Niche. Does this define passion? We are told that if we are passionate about something we will go all out to acquire it.

Let us pause to explore Bryant's behavior towards Sally, the girl who has just moved in next door, on whom he is quickly developing a crush. He may start showing episodes of kindness to Sally which may continue till Sally reciprocates, if she is interested, eventually those two become friends, as their vibrational energies come into alignment. Their emotional alignment will encourage increments which will allow drift along the emotional positioning system towards the zone of happiness. As time continues the further evolution within the happiness zone continues if their vibrational energies remain in alignment. The spirit is positively fed by this emotional alignment which will massage the mindset and encourage the behavior manifested by the body. This may morph into a strong friendship or even a relationship. Using this understanding of how the emotions impact the spirit and massages our mindset which eventually manifests in our behavior leads to a better understanding of marital disharmony and breakdown. Simply put, marital disharmony and breakdown is the result of breakage in the alignment of the vibrational energies in couples. As an individual you have a specific vibrational energy, you meet someone whose vibrational energy aligns with yours and that gives the feeling of safety, you feel sufficiently safe or inquisitive to want to peep into that other person's vibrations, how (s)he thinks, how (s)he behaves in a particular circumstance etc. If there is some emotional alignment then that will create a harmonious partnership, bearing in mind that you are both separate individuals with different vibrations. Hence once this vibrational alignment starts to move out of alignment, cracks develop. Cracks are of three stages. Stage 1 or short cracks, Stage 2 or long cracks and stage 3 complete fracture. The fracture mechanism theory, addressing the rupture of a solid body defines stages of crack development. The fracturing process is described as a progressive failure that usually consists of three stages;(1) crack initiation, (2) slow crack growth and (3) rapid crack propagation. If not recognized and addressed the fissure gets wider and eventually a fracture results. Marriage counsellors continue to advise that couples reflect on prior happy moments, what they are almost innocuously implying may be unknowingly, is revisiting a time when the vibrations between the couple were aligned. Their success in saving a marriage is dependent on the stage in the development of the crack. At the point of crack initiation and at varying locations along the development in the slow growth of the crack, a band aid like approach may be sufficient to obtain realignment, but the further along the cracking process the more difficult it is to obtain realignment. Unfortunately, many a counsellor may not necessarily appreciate this and use the same bland band aid approach in trying to repair the crack, failure is the usual result. Better appreciation of the position along the cracking processes a couple is, may define the appropriate strategy to be used and lead to better success. It is felt that if we can get there, we may be better positioned to apply more effective resolution strategies.

Wellbeing

Dr. Seligman, the father of the positive psychology movement, wrote that happiness is only one component of a sense of overall well-being. Well-being to him is composed of five components:

1. Positive emotion - this encompasses all positive feelings e.g. Joy, comfort, and pleasure.

2. Engagement - this relates to the depth to which you are absorbed in a subject.

3. Positive Relationships - relationships with whom you can share your highs and lows.

4. Meaning - relates to the sense of belonging or serving something greater than oneself.

5. Accomplishment - associated with the process in acquiring as opposed to the acquisition.

Happiness and well-being are not goals per se; they are more of a process, a journey if you will. They are not a fixed acquisition they more aptly define the process one goes through to acquire the object. Happiness therefore becomes an ongoing process. There is good evidence that optimism and happiness coexist, and both lead to healthier, more successful, and more fulfilling lives, a mirror of the process in growing into your excellence and a testament that marriage or relationships requires continuous effort to maintain them and even more effort to grow them.

We must recognize that it takes effort to improve our emotional lives, and that the effort does make a difference. Now that we have that piece of the puzzle in place, let us move on to examining the environments in which your spirit will remain nourished and therefore flourish!

Reflection:

What is the human spirit?

How can you nourish the human spirit?

What does the emotional Guidance system tell you?

How does doubt influence your actions?

Is happiness an emotion?

How can one explain the breakdown in a relationship?

How can your wellbeing be assured?

_____

_____

_____

_____

_____

_____

_____

_____

_____

_____

_____

_____

Chapter 16: Nurturing Your spirit

"The best way to cheer yourself up is to try to cheer somebody else up." —
Mark Twain

Steps

In attempting to obtain the best and safest environment in which
to nurture your spirit, you will doubtlessly meet some negative people
along your path. To ensure that your spirit is appropriately nourished, let
us explore ways in which you can deal with the negative ones we
encounter along the highway of life including within ourselves parading
as our ego.

Negative people

Unfortunately, negative people seem talented at reducing any
progress which you have made, in almost any sphere of your life. It is
therefore palpably important to be capable of addressing these people to
sustain your happiness and well-being and so add years to your life and
life to your years while you grow into your excellence. Allow me to suggest
a stepwise process to reduce the input from the negative ones with whom
you may come into contact.

Step 1: Cultivate boundaries, never seek advice from a negative
person. Interestingly, these people are always willing and ready to offer
advice, even if that advice is unsolicited. Be prepared to establish
boundaries, even if you may be unfamiliar with the individual offering the
advice, do a quick assessment of where that person is in life and determine

if that is where you see yourself going, if the answer is no, then discard the advice without a second thought.

Step 2: Accept them for who they are and make an informed decision about how much you want or need them in your life. You need to determine the significance of these people in your life, what do they contribute to your growth, your mindset, or your personality. You may realize that they make a light contribution to your mood or your exercise program and as such you only engage them in these activities, maybe sharing a joke or maybe going to the gym with them but outside of those entities you do not consider them as 'your friends' with whom you spend quality time or with whom you engage in meaningful discussions. In other words, you have categories of friendships or friends for occasions. For example, as a medical doctor, I have been amazed by the offerings of some folks. I was introduced to a fraudster masquerading as a project manager who offered to train me to speak publicly at a cost. Our paths quickly changed direction with mine going in the opposite direction from his. One must therefore be cautious of those who are making offers that they cannot deliver. You may be better positioned to deliver what they seek to deliver to you, but they first try to destroy your confidence.

Step 3: Avoid trying to get caught in the game of trying to win one against a negative person. For example, a person complaining about the behavior of his teenage son, don't try to outdo her by claiming that your own son has a drug issue. If you find yourself doing this, try to nip it before it starts to fester.

Step 4: Be an adult. If a negative person needs support or reassurance give it to them if they need to be right let them be right. Try to avoid arguments with a negative person because they will win every time, bringing you down to their level.

Step 5: Recognize and know that it is alright to walk away from a negative person. Be prepared to do so even if they are family members, though this may be initially difficult, but by gradually creating distance between yourself and that person you will achieve the desired goal.

Step 6: If you are the boss and an employee is always negative, recognize that this attitude could have an impact on the work environment, affecting productivity and employee morale. Be prepared to address this even if it means terminating the employee. As is frequently said, one bad apple spoils the whole lot, don't allow one negative person to destroy your business. Remember the environment can influence your spirit which can impact your mindset and create difficulty in nurturing your growth.

Step 7: You are all about creating positivity, so your effort should be focused on building a network of people with spirits in the happy zone of the emotional positioning system, this will positively impact mindsets which will be an ideal environment for nourishing your spirit.

These suggestions, I hear you say, address only negativity that is outside of your person, what about that which is internal?

Internal Negativity

We have established that negativity irrespective of its source is not healthy for the spirit in that it leads to affecting our position on the emotional positioning system and so adversely affects the nourishment of our spirit with the result that we move down the emotional positioning system. Yet we learn of our ego, a phenomenon designed to keep us rational and potentially protect us.

This tends to chime in when attempting to explore the unknown. Remember the internal criticism that you experienced when trying to embark on anything different? Your impression of yourself is questioned, your competence is questioned, you may be accused of being selfish, because of the need for time to develop your dream etc. internal criticism can be harsh enough to create uncertainty leading to doubt. This doubt starves the spirit causing the individual to occupy a relatively lower position on the EPS. Thus, internal negativity can affect your spirit in the same manner as external criticism. One will expect internal criticism probably because of the need to be perfect, an unachievable ideal. Author Ray Bradbury understands the role played by our internal critic; he advises us that we 'should not think'. He claims that thinking is the enemy of creativity. It's self-conscious, and anything self-conscious is lousy. You can't try to do things; you simply must do things. I don't subscribe to this teaching, as a universal principle. The moment determines how much thought can be allowed. Our physiology also dictates how we respond to an event. We have all been schooled that in the face of an imminent threat our response is to fight or run away (the fight or flight phenomenon) this response is designed to keep us safe, there is however a third response

185

which we hear very little off, but we see practiced repeatedly, particularly among lower members in the animal kingdom. In some cases that phenomenon is further exacerbated by these organisms letting off smelly fumes to further convince the predator that they are dead and rotting. This response tends to be seen in cases where a predator is attacking prey. Should this phenomenon be practiced by humans? The response is simple, it depends on the scenario. If for example, you are being attacked by a brown or grizzly bear, the option of running may not be appropriate, fighting may be less than ideal cause you will invariably emerge on the wrong end, but if you choose to freeze, the bear may leave you alone. This practice though should not be considered appropriate when facing an attack by any other bear. Most definitely, not a polar bear. This phenomenon, called the freeze is employed when either trying to run away or fighting does not afford us adequate protection, so animals assume the posture of death.

Other authors have advised that we should jump and develop our wings on the way down. Inherent in this statement is that there may be a dive before growth. It will require belief, commitment, and patience. How does growth occur? I hear you ask. To respond, we must appreciate the words of James Baldwin who famously said, not everything that is faced can be changed. But nothing can be changed until it is faced. This is necessary for growth to occur. Growth though is a painful experience. Imagine that you are trying to develop your biceps (the muscle at the front of your arm between the front of your elbow and the front of your shoulder. To do this you join a gym at which you engage in resistance training exercises. During exercise sessions you push yourself to the limit.

Following your work out, you feel the pains in your arms, but you keep pushing, eventually the bulge from the biceps becomes more prominent. Growth with pain is made possible with persistence. To grow our spirit, we may need to withstand resistance from both within and without. It requires us to experience pain, self-doubt, self-criticism, as well as criticism from external sources, which as noted can be very harsh. Synonymous with growth is strength. The result is we become more powerful. Could it be the ego's attempt to prevent us from exploring paths unknown based on the negative emotion of fear? Fearful that we may become too powerful? This may well be. Consider that you have developed a small cake baking business at home. As word gets out your business seems to be flourishing; you start thinking of expanding your business. You wish to have more space you are thinking of renting a unit and employing some help. Instantly the resistance starts questioning your ability and the practicability of your thoughts. You listen and cave into the negativity. On the contrary, you appreciate the internal resistance, but through whichever means you choose, you overcome this negative self-talk and proceed with your dream. With effort and commitment, you push on through, your business grows, and you increase your reach, thus becoming more powerful. You now have employees, you have improved management skills, you are better known etc., all a reflection of power. Could it be that the role played by negativism whether externally or internally is predicated on fear (a negative emotion). Fear that you grow and become too powerful. Growth as stated above is not without pain. Are negative forces whether they arise from internal or external factors designed to rob you of your power?

You are designed to be a happy human being! As we have discussed in the previous chapter your emotions indicate if your spirit is being adequately nourished. Your spirit will also guide you towards environments that will provide the best nourishment and prevent you from falling prey to negative emotions. The adage "Birds of a feather flock together" can be applied here. Abraham-Hicks teaches us, your spirit will seek out elements which have the same vibration as your own. You may not realize it, but you have probably already experienced it.

Have you ever been in the company of someone, and you just don't jive with them, even though you cannot find anything wrong with them per se? Or perhaps you have been at a gathering or event and have the desire to leave even though there really isn't anything wrong. Upon entering you felt good and were looking forward to enjoying yourself but shortly after you stepped into the room something felt uncomfortable and you wanted to leave. This is the reaction of your spirit meeting energetic vibrations that don't align. Your spirit wants to be in the company of people whose spirit is aligned with your own because it facilitates your happiness! Be mindful that as you continue to work on adding years to your life and life to your years and grow into your excellence, you may find your spirit not vibrating on the same plane as some people who have usually felt close to you. If your vibrational alignment shifts, so may your desire to be around particular people. Be aware of this phenomenon.

Natural Laws and the Law of Attraction

Permit me to revisit the law of attraction.

Natural laws are objective, universal, and exist independently outside of general human understanding and society at large. Just as morality (what we view as right and wrong) is applied to everyone, so are the natural laws. Over the years, the natural laws have been studied and written about by scholars. There is one law, in particular, that is directly associated with the creation of the appropriate environment that ensures that your vibrations are in alignment. When your vibrations are appropriately aligned as we have seen above it facilitates appropriate movement along the EGS. Your spirit is then nourished, and your emotions may reach an appropriate level on the EGS, that is moving towards level 1. The natural law is referred to as, 'The Law of Attraction.'

A simple workable definition for the law of attraction is referenced in Abraham-Hicks's teachings as "that which is like unto itself is drawn". In other words, like attracts like, and positive or negative thoughts may bring positive or negative experiences into your life. This may seem to have manifested itself time and time again in our lives, and we have accepted it for what it is. But is it true? Does it work on some occasions but not others? Could there be another component to this law that is needed to make it true in your life?

I think the law as stated may be an oversimplification and lacks a key element before it can be appreciated as a natural law which works every time. The law is not as simple as stated. There is a **bridge** needed to attach or draw like to like. Think of two identical pieces of metal lying

189

side by side. They are the same, yet they exist as two separate items. But by magnetizing one, the pieces of metal would be magnetically attracted to each other and stick together. This magnetization is the bridge attracting like to like. Some among you may quickly and rightfully argue that this phenomenon is only seen in metallic substances and substances which can be magnetized. Does this law apply to pieces of lumber? Of course, lumber cannot be magnetized but we can get lumber sticking to each other by applying a bridge, be it glue, nails, or some other bridging entity. The message here is simply to get like to adhere, there is need for a bridge. Since attraction is not always evident, between identical objects consideration should be given to renaming the law of attraction to the law of bridging. Simply put, the Law of Attraction claims that like attracts like. This does not seem to be universally applicable. There is always a need for a bridge. Once that bridge is present like can adhere to like more efficiently than like to unlike. The law of attraction is a catchier name and may not be changed but as stated it can be misleading. In your own life, this sort of bridging energy is necessary when working with and applying the Law of Attraction. In our human form, this magnetization is our **FOCUS**, described above as our passion, some may say **COMMITMENT**. Commitment you will agree drives and defines our focus.

The required level of focus is reflected in a common saying by Les Brown who claims that if you want something bad enough you will go out and fight for it, you will work day and night for it, you will give up your time, your peace and sleep for it, If all that you dream and scheme is about it….with the help of God you will get it. This reflects intense focus, commitment, and passion if you will. This is described as the FLOW by Psychologist Dr Mihaly Csikszentmihalyi, one of the founders of the positive psychology movement. Dr Csikszentmihalyi describes six key features of the **FLOW**.

The Flow

1. It involves intense focused concentration on the present moment.

2. Causes action and awareness to merge.

3. There is a loss of self – consciousness, this may lead to a temporary loss of sensations such as hunger and pain.

4. There is a strong sense of personal control.

5. You lose track of time.

6. The activity is pleasurable or rewarding, regardless of the potential goal or outcome.

Flow he contends can occur because of both professional and leisure activities. There is increasing evidence that people who are routinely able to attain a state of **FLOW** are happier overall.

Many have attempted to unravel this apparent puzzle, and several have hinted to the failure of this supposedly natural law, the law of attraction, since it occasionally fails to withstand scrutiny. We have mentioned the saying "what you conceive and believe, you can achieve". Simply conceiving is not sufficient, the element of belief becomes a necessary ingredient, the "magnetizer" if you will. The depth of our belief determines our focus and whether the Law of attraction will be activated. Therefore, the law of attraction fails to exist without the appropriate magnetization or focus. The focus of your thoughts will magnetize and attract other similar (like) thoughts and feelings. These magnetized aspects will also attract to you anything that is on the same vibration. Please be mindful that this is applied as always to thoughts good or bad. You must be aware of how you are feeling and what thoughts are bringing you into these emotional states, as you will attract what you are feeling and thinking based on the degree of energy or focus you place on the feeling or thoughts. You want to ensure your focus is appropriate so that it will serve you, attracting that which you desire!

Interestingly the role of magnetization is not new and has long been practiced in the Christian community. Faith in the bible is defined as the assurance of things hoped for, the evidence of things not seen. As the bible says several times, ask and it shall be given. However, it is the faith that one has which is seen as magnetizing this "ask" and the gifts from God. This is stated most clearly in the new living translation bible in Mathews chapter: 21 and verse 22; you can pray for anything, and if you have faith, you will receive it. Most commonly, faith is shown in the act of prayer. Praying can be seen as the act of requesting.

Your faith brings into focus that for which you ask. Evidence of the law of attraction and focus can be seen in this scenario.

Case in point, you have just bought a new car, and you have now started to see more and more cars on the road like the one you just bought. Do you believe that it is because of the Law of Attraction that your new car simply attracts these other cars which were hardly noticeable before you purchased your new car? Is it that since you bought your new car everybody has now bought and is driving the very same vehicle that you bought? Surely, you will agree that's not a rational way to think about it. But a more reasonable lens to see this through is that since your focus has now changed, you are now noticing cars like yours as you drive. So, the question then becomes how do you create the bridge from thought to reality in your own life?

Reflection:

Can I remember a time where the company I was in made me feel "off" or uneasy?

How did it make me feel when I didn't leave?

What are my thoughts on the Law of Attraction?

Can I think of something right now that I have been trying to manifest but have not been putting in the work or focus which is required to magnetize it and attract it to me?

_____

_____

_____

_____

_____

_____

_____

_____

_____

_____

This aspect of your spirit continues to be a fascinating and rich part of your adding years to your life and life to your years while you grow into your excellence. It can all seem so simple and yet so complicated. Now that you understand the law of attraction and how through your own focus, you can make it a working part of your life, let's go back to discussing your Emotional Guidance System (EGS). Together with your comprehension of the law of attraction and your EGS, we can begin exploring how things outside of yourself may impact your spirit. Remember that all these aspects are working closely together to revive your spirit and must be in place to bring more years to your life and life to your years while accompanying you in your growth into your excellence.

Chapter 17: Impact on Our Spirit

"We have nothing to fear but fear itself." – Franklin D. Roosevelt

Understanding the Spirit

Your spirit is designed to keep you comfortable and happy in your life. Your spirit wants to support you and be an advocate for you in times of need. It is beautifully intertwined with your emotions. Your emotions can act as an indicator of the state of your spirit and if you are in line with the higher vibrations of your potential.

If something or someone impacts you emotionally, your spirit will be impacted. This may look like unsolicited advice, inappropriate comments, a sudden loss, or a yearning for the beauty of the forest, etc. Without warning these are things that will trigger your emotions. The ways in which your spirit may be impacted are varied and can occur at any time of your day. To ensure you have control and benefit from this, acquiring the advantage it affords you, let us again look to your Emotional Guidance System. Let's further explore how you can empower yourself in aiding your spirit to be safeguarded from circumstances that may impact you.

Revisiting the Emotional Guidance System (EGS)

A quick reminder that your EGS has two terminals and a plethora of emotions in between. You can determine where you are and where you are headed (higher or lower vibrational state) based on movements and changes in your emotions. As previously compared, our EGS is like an internal GPS.

GPS systems only work because of the input with from external factors such as traffic, road closures etc. its internal circuitry. A GPS system collects data from multiple external sources so that it may guide you to your destination as quickly and efficiently as possible. Similarly, the emotions that your EGS is founded on will undoubtedly be impacted by Both outside and internal sources, therefore directing your EGS directions. You are either heading to bright and joyful emotions or continuing down through negative emotions. In both the GPS and EGS systems, what is always needed is a pilot. This is **you**. You have the power within you to ensure your EGS is being steered in the right direction.

The comparison of the EGS to a standard GPS is apt. With the GPS, the only instruction required is where you want to go. You may streamline your route by asking the GPS to use the quickest available route, and to avoid traffic etc. With the EGS, you can request anything from the universe and allow your spirit to fine tune its delivery. We recognize that the EGS has only two poles which makes it very user friendly. You guide the direction of the flow with your emotions. I encourage you to exercise emotional control.

When external factors begin affecting your emotions, it is necessary to understand how they are engaging with your belief system or if they are just fleeting thoughts. Thoughts can be either acute or chronic thoughts. While your acute thoughts are ones that just seem to pop up and leave as quickly as they came, Chronic thoughts are ones that are constantly present or that are long standing, and thus create your belief systems. The impact of external factors on our thoughts will always be determined by you. For you to have a clear understanding of this and how it impacts you, let's look at a situation where the acute and chronic thought systems come into play. Remember, your attention to the matter enhances your focus and therefore magnetizes your goals and desires, enhancing the receipt of both your goals and desires.

The EGS at Work

Let's dive into a relatable example of how your thoughts and the EGS can work for you or against you. The key is you must be willing to work with managing your belief system, your mindset, if you will through the management of your spirit.

Lisa is morbidly obese and has been trying to lose weight for some time. She has tried at least three different weight loss programs with no success. Because of these failures Lisa begins harboring negative thoughts that diets do not work. She begins to develop a belief system around diets. Lisa's friend introduces her to a new diet plan that she has been trying for 3 months with noticeable plausible results. After some encouragement from her friend, Lisa decides to try this new diet plan even though she now holds a strong belief that diets don't work, and she does not expect to be successful.

Lisa's chronic thoughts and emotions around diets have created a belief that this diet will not work. How is this diet expected to work? Remember, Lisa is living in a vibration of believing that it won't? Lisa's thoughts ("diets don't work") and her desires ("I want to lose weight with this diet plan") don't match up! If they are not synchronized, based on what we know with how the EGS works and how the Law of Attraction is activated through magnetization, focus; Lisa is expected to continue to fail with this new diet plan. Along the EGS path, Lisa's emotion is one of doubt, she will continue to fail at dieting. The magnetization in this case is based on Lisa's chronic thoughts, her focus, that diets don't work, an element of internal negativity. It is her belief and since she believes that diets don't work, her focus will draw thoughts and behaviors to her magnetized belief system ensuring that this diet plan does not work.

Lisa's actions will remain in line with her beliefs that diets do not work. If portion control is in question, she is much more likely to not adhere to her diet's guidelines. To her, it is foolish to make the sacrifice by controlling her portion sizes when she knows the diet won't work. She will attract thoughts and behaviors which will ensure that this diet will fail – the law of attraction in action. When she checks her weight and has gained a few pounds because of not following her diet guidelines, she will then have demonstrated the workings of the law of attraction and find herself falling further down her EGS. In this example, Lisa has asked the Universe to facilitate her weight loss (acute thoughts) but because her acute thoughts were not synchronous with her belief system ("diets don't work," chronic thoughts,) she was not prepared to receive her gift of weight management.

The universe will give that for which you seek if your belief system (chronic thoughts) and acute thoughts are in alignment. You must be prepared to receive that for which you asked. Factors which activate opposing vibrations to your desires will lead to a failure in your receiving your desire. Your focus and the resultant magnetization will shift your vibrations in the direction of your focus, in this example, diets don't work. The result is the fulfillment of your belief, your focus, diets don't work. The vibrations of your chronic thoughts are opposed by the vibrations of your acute thoughts with the result that your chronic thoughts vibrations override the acute thoughts leading to your failure in acquiring that which you requested, the product of your acute thoughts. Your acute thoughts are always your request, and your chronic thoughts are your belief system. The interplay between your acute and chronic thoughts will prevent you from acquiring what you desire in life unless they are in alignment. Take immediate responsibility for what you are and are not bringing into your world. Begin examining different areas of your life and see if you have some acute thoughts in play that don't seem to be getting you anywhere.

Dig deep and notice if you have beliefs in different areas that are preventing you from moving forward and moving up in your EGS towards more joy and happiness. You must remove the discord between your desire (acute thoughts) and your belief (chronic thoughts). As we have mentioned, once you have recognized that your chronic and acute thoughts are not congruent, it is then time to clarify what you need and hence enhance your focus, which may bring you into the '**FLOW**'; deep focus and concentration, thus facilitating your movement ahead. Remove distractions and work on ensuring that your desire (acute thoughts) is in line with your goal (chronic thoughts). The Universe will activate the law of attraction, to support your chronic thoughts and deliver your goal to you.

Reflection:

When have my chronic thoughts (or belief system) taken me further away from a goal I desire?

Can I see a direct correlation in my life when my acute thoughts and chronic thoughts were not aligned and therefore prevented me from achieving my goal?

Reflect on a time in your life when you asked the universe for something, for example money to pay your utility bill. You have no idea where the money is coming from, but you are focused on acquiring the money. Has the universe delivered the money to you?

_____

_____

_____

_____

_____

_____

_____

Chapter 18: Belief and Faith

The Impact of Belief

In our example with Lisa, if she embarked on the new weight loss plan harboring thoughts such as "I know this works and I have seen great results in my friend", she would be starting out from a great place because her chronic thoughts would be strong, and she would be focused on the positive. She would start believing that since it worked for her friend, she was determined to make it work for her. Lisa would be focused on bringing herself in line with her goal. She would heighten her focus, leading to magnetization and activation of the law of attraction which would attract factors which when employed by Lisa would allow her to obtain her goal. She will focus on how the program will work if she follows it and this will magnetize more positive thoughts to her. Lisa would then begin seeing the fruits of her labor which would then cause her to feel better about herself and inspire her to stay on a disciplined track with the new diet. Her emotions would shift causing her to get higher on the EGS and closer towards reaping the fruits of her desire. It is simple but conscious effort, commitment, patience, and focus are necessary.

Faith and the EGS

This is how faith works in activating the law of attraction. What you think of will attract its vibration towards you. You must trust that this is the case. You must believe that even though you cannot see it now, you will achieve it. Faith is that focus necessary to magnetize your desire so

201

that you can achieve your goal. You have faith in the process, and you have faith in the future outcome. As you continue to climb higher on your own EGS, you feel a sense of relief and a willingness to keep believing.

Reflection:

Can I think of an example where I truly believed in something and was able to climb higher on my EGS and in turn attract what I wanted towards me?

How does it make me feel to have faith and be willing to keep trying?

What stands in the way of my greatness?

_____

_____

_____

_____

_____

_____

_____

_____

When trying to create change in your life, your role is to constantly reach for a feeling of improvement. You can actively cultivate tools to facilitate your positivity, thereby minimizing the effects of negativity on your spirit. Interestingly, when you are relaxed, your brain waves, muscles, heart rate, even breathing and all your bodily processes are in a calm state but these change and become more excitable as you become agitated. Experts have advised that through a sort of biofeedback mechanism you should attempt to use information on the biological processes in your body to help train yourself into a positive mental and physical state.

This may involve focusing on the biological process of your own breathing and may facilitate a sort of feedback loop leading to a calmer you. Journaling may allow for the development of new skills and practices which promote happiness and well-being. Dr Siegel contends that the act of writing down our stories activates the narrator's function in our minds allowing us to process the event fully and thereby prevent it from provoking current unexpected physical and emotional responses. Journaling allows us to assimilate our past and allows us to assess it. This allows us to overcome trauma, adversity, and finally, through meditation we can train our brain to go to a peaceful, happy or relaxed state and thereby stave off an agitated state.

By employing these three entities or combinations of these entities, we can develop skills to allow us to cope with the vicissitudes of daily life and thereby facilitate our happiness and sense of well-being.

Coping Mechanisms

The American poet, Langston Hughes, reminds us in his poem *Mother to Son,* that "...life is no crystal stair, there are tacks in it, splinters, board torn up and places with no carpets on the floor, bare, ... "

Martin Luther King Jr chided us that it is only when it is dark enough can we see the stars. So, we know that despite our efforts, there will be challenges, and we will need to find coping mechanisms if we are to keep going forward. It is easy to stay positive and emotionally happy when times are good but when things go wrong our coping strategies will be tested. It is in this scenario that familiarity with and understanding of the BMS ecosystem and its principles rises to the fore and liberates you from the clutches of the malaise.

Our sense of purpose and our social connections can prove dramatically helpful to our physical well-being. It is true we mentioned in section one about the benefits of healthy eating, exercising, temperance, sunlight, water, rest, and air. These are essential elements in maintaining a healthy physical body, but it takes more to be healthy. Too often we seem to show reduced attention to our emotional health, and growth, which is just as important as our physical health, if we are to enjoy the addition of years to our life and life to our years, while allowing you to grow into your excellence. As reflected on the EGS, if our emotional health is appropriately cared for, we can enjoy the fruits of the spirit with its remarkable attributes.

The EGS will indicate to us the status of our emotional health. If your emotional state is not predominantly at the upper levels of your EGS, then we need to address this; otherwise, your physical health will be adversely affected. As indicated above, the upper levels of the EGS are synonymous with a positive or growth mind set. The literature is replete with the benefits to your physical, mental, and spiritual health and the contribution this makes to adding years to your life and life to your years. This also facilitates your growth into your excellence. The development of a positive mindset which is integrally related to an elevated positioning on the EGS, has overall health benefits and is the crux of the BMS ecosystem.

Try to determine why you are in an unsatisfactory emotional state. Is there a lack of meaning in your day-to-day life or is your circle of socialization too small, lacks variety or interest? If so, try new activities. This will allow you to establish new contacts, keep active and generate interest in your life. Reach out to classmates, hear their stories, reminisce on school days, have a laugh, start a social media group.... Being a part of a community has immeasurable benefits, not least of all Catharsis.

If the unsatisfactory emotional state is the result of interpersonal conflicts, set boundaries. Avoid spending time with the person with whom there is a conflict. Alternatively, improving your communication with that individual by becoming more empathetic and a more active listener could help to reduce the conflict which would be mutually beneficial.

If the cause of your unsatisfactory emotional state is because of a change in your life, be it major physical injury, a divorce or even the death of a family member, cognitive flexibility will help you to cope. Simply put, it is a way of thinking and seeing things in a different way. For example, maybe if you are going through a divorce. Cognitive flexibility may involve you thinking about the positive benefits of divorce. In the case of the death of a family member, being able to reminisce on the good times you have had with that person and the fact that your life was more fulfilled for having them around will most definitely help you to cope. Falling back on your signature strengths (the abilities that contribute to our happiness and well-being and that come relatively easy to us) will prove to be a useful ally when coping with bad news.

You will know that you are moving in the right direction by a drift in your emotions toward happier emotions on the EGS. The results will be bearing the fruits of the spirit that you seek. It is always there for the taking. But as discussed, I urge you to not allow your old beliefs to get in the way. Be prepared to get out of your own way and **BE THANKFUL**. This is about your life now. This is about your revival! You have the power to create a life filled with joy and vitality. I believe in you!

Reflection:

How can belief affect our EGS?

Does faith have any impact on our EGS?

List five coping mechanisms that you revert to in order to influence your EGS.

_____

_____

_____

_____

_____

_____

_____

_____

Chapter 19: Stress Management

Defining Stress

Stress is more than a feeling or a single occurrence. Rather, it is a cycle with several steps, it starts with an event which galvanizes you into action from the resting state and ends when you have overcome the threat, and you are now safe. Stress is therefore designed to protect you.

Types of Stress

Fear/Grief/Depression/Despair/Powerlessness/Stress, occupies the lowest pole on the EGS, since this is not a healthy place to be we will explore how we can elevate ourselves from this, the nadir of our emotional positioning system (EPS). Stress describes our body's response to pressure or a stressful situation. Our body's response is to protect us and keep us safe in the face of a pressure situation or threat. When threatened by a predator, the ensuing stress allows us to quickly analyze the situation and determine our options for self-protection. Do we have enough time to run away to safety or what are our chances if we were to stand and fight. To give us the necessary tools we need, at least the naturally occurring substances called stress hormones are released into our circulation which allows us to react appropriately. The stress hormones of which I speak are adrenalin and cortisol. This leads to a cascade of interactions leading to the phenomenon of the fight or flight response. In lower animals, there is a third response we see, the freeze, in which animals faced with an overwhelming threat which they are unable to fight off, or run away from, may feign death, a phenomenon called the freeze, a sort of tonic, highly activated state of immobility. This distracts the predator, giving the prey time to escape. Though this practice is not advisable in human beings, it is successful if attacked by a brown bear. This response to immediate stress is the triple F response, fight, flight, and freeze. This response is identified when in immediate danger, hence distinguishing acute stress from chronic stress. In chronic stress, the presentation may not be as dramatic, but the physiological exposure to the stress hormones still exists and our bodies remain internally bathed by these stress juices. There are two types of stress (a) acute which describes a case of imminent danger evoking the 3 F response (Fight, Flight, or Freeze) and (b) a less dramatic event which evokes similar responses, but it is continuous.

The Stress Cycle

Medical researcher, A.Z. Reznick outlines the stress cycle as follows (a) A resting state (that is before the threat), (b) Tension and strain phase (that is on perception of the threat) the initial response to a stressor that triggers the fight or flight reaction as the body is prepared for action, (c) the response phase, (That describes how you respond to the threat, it may be an active or passive response) and (d) the relief phase, (which is both physiological and psychological) and describes the phase in which the body and mind return to the resting state after the stressor is removed or resolved.

The stress cycle describes a natural sequence of steps which your body encounters when dealing with stress. Over time your body has developed a mechanism comprised of three general steps to help it to respond to stress. These three steps are alarm, resistance, and exhaustion.

Alarm tends to be most pronounced in the face of an acute stressor. For example, you are being attacked by an aggressive wild animal. The sight of the threat causes your body to be flooded with stress hormones which allows you to quickly evaluate the scenario and to decide the safest way in which to respond which falls into one of the three F's (a) fight if you can overcome your attacker and it's safe to do so. (b) You may run away if you are able, not always possible and (c)If you are unable to fight or run away, pretending to be dead called the freeze, is the third option. An act commonly seen in lower animals. In doing so, the predator tends to relax giving the prey an opportunity to escape.

Is Stress Management Important?

When exposed to stress, the body's stress response is triggered. This leads to an increase in the heart rate, increased rate of breathing, deviation of blood from organs which are less involved in helping us to fight or runaway and increasing the supply of blood to our skeletal muscles. This response is expected to last for only a short period before you recover and continue your normal activity. Sometimes though this stress is constant, you never give yourself time to recover. If the cycle persists and continues indefinitely, you develop chronic stress. There is an increased dumping of glucose or our body's energy currency into our blood stream. This occurs irrespective of our response, whether we run, fight or freeze.

Despite the changes our body undergoes when exposed to stress, it is designed to protect us, all three responses, fight, flight, and freeze are reflexes designed to protect us. The response to acute stress is therefore protective. Chronic stress though is not and can lead to health problems, such as cardiovascular disease, diabetes, stokes, mental illnesses and even some types of cancers, it may also manifest with disturbed sleep, weight gain or weight loss, avoidance of self-care, poor mood, social isolation, and negative self-talk.

Chronic stress can be triggered by several factors, among them are (a) work related such as feeling pressure at work, unemployment, or retirement, (b) family or relationship issues, divorce or caring for someone, (c) Financial problems- unexpected bills or burrowing money and (d) health – illness, injury, or bereavement. Since stress is ubiquitous and inevitable with punitive sequelae every effort must be made to manage it appropriately.

Chronic Stress

As seen above the stress response is designed to protect and is expected to be a brief response. Once the initial threat subsides, the stress response is reduced. The level of the stress juices (hormones), fall off, the blood pressure and heart rate move towards normalcy, the body begins the recovery process but remains on high alert till the stressful event is no longer an issue.

If the stressor is chronic such as a demanding job, an unhappy relationship, a concern with your finances, your body remains in a state of heightened alert and the stress hormones remain high.

To cope, your body makes several adjustments which may not be healthy, you may experience poor sleep, your ability to concentrate may be negatively impacted and your mood may be low. This can adversely impact your entire being. The impact of stress is so pronounced that it is the lowest emotion on the emotional positioning system. Chronic stress management is integral to our wellbeing if we are to grow into excellence. Failure to manage chronic Stress leads to exhaustion.

Exhaustion and its Sequelae

Persistent stress coupled with the inability to complete the stress cycle causes the body to repeat the stress response, which will cause our body to remain in a state of high alert, the result is long-term health issues such as fatigue, anxiety, depression, stomach ulcers and mental burnout. We aim to break free from the stress cycle by identifying healthy coping mechanisms and introducing them into our lives.

The 6R stress busting Syndicate

These chronic stress triggers are more common than we care to admit. Chronic stress, unlike its acute counterpart, is not protective and adversely affects our overall physical as well as mental health. It is this stress we need to manage effectively or else the diseases listed above can affect us. It is here that we use the 6R Stress busting Syndicate to effectively manage the stress. This stress buster syndicate is composed of the Review, empowered by the P.E.E.L back tool kit, Here the aim is to determine the underlying cause. In the Remove phase empowered by the euthanasia effect, we aim to rip away the cause of the stress. The regeneration then becomes necessary, since we know that nature abhors

212

an empty space, we will therefore replace the space created by the removal of the stress by using the new C.A.R.E model. After we replace the stressor using the new care model, We then reset the T.R.A.P which kept us stressed, this phase is the Reserve phase, to ensure the replacement is not fleeting, We will be relieved as the result of our intervention allows the client to go through the M.O.R.P.H motivator process and finally the emerging with the big L.I.G.H.T.E.D release thus ensuring that (s)he is free from stress. This 6R stress busting syndicate is a progressive process which must be followed systematically to obtain the best result.

You can learn more about the 6R Stress busting syndicate for the management of Stress as taught by the Philburn academy.

Reflection:

How many types of stress are you familiar with?

Can stress ever be good?

If stress is good, why is it necessary to try to manage it?

What are the elements of the 6R stress busting syndicate?

What is the 6R stress busting syndicate designed to achieve?

Are you more productive when stressed?

What are stress juices?

_____

_____

_____

_____

_____

_____

_____

_____

_____

_____

Chapter 20: Journaling – The Focus Intensifier

"Journal writing is a voyage to the interior." – Christina Baldwin

Journaling

What is Journaling? I hear you ask. Simply put, it is what the name implies, it involves creating a document of your thoughts, feelings, and experiences daily. This is also described as scripting. It is not always a written article; it can be a photographic collection with a few words next to the picture. Journaling has many benefits, among which are the management of stress and anxiety. It can also help you to place in order your worries, concerns, and problems. Symptoms of both your physical and mental health are recognized, the result is you become aware of your various triggers, and this can allow you to develop coping strategies.

The journaling process may take the form of a written story, it may be short notes, or even a single word may be used to describe your thoughts, feelings, and experiences.

It is advisable that you start your journal with an expression of gratitude to God or some may say to the universe. Journaling can aid you in the management and change of your self-talk. Since writing gives an opportunity to reflect, your will identify the way you talk to yourself. Negative self-talk will be identified and changed to positive ones. The result is incremental movement up the ECS and this thus helps you to feel better about yourself. Gradually you will get to know yourself better, it acts as a mirror to your inner self. Journaling also helps with your mental health and there is evidence that it improves your physical health. Journaling strengthens the immune system and reduces the time it takes to recover from sickness and injury. Baikie and Wilhelm (2005) came to a similar conclusion from their study. Eatough (2021) indicates that writing down your goals helps you to achieve them. This can be explained by the act of writing allowing increase focus, thus providing the magnetization necessary for the law of Attraction to be activated and manifested.

There is no specific time to start journaling. 5-10 minutes at any time of the day would be appropriate. The individual determines the time most convenient to them. Many proponents advise that Journaling be practiced as you rise from bed in the morning. Done this way, it ensures you start your day with an organized plan and calmness. Others prefer to do it at the end of their workday or school day. This allows them to reflect on the events of the day, their thoughts, feelings, and experiences, especially the challenging experiences. One would also recommend that Journaling is done at the same time daily. If life gets in the way of allowing you to do journaling daily, don't place undue pressure on yourself, you may just resume the following day. Journaling should preferably be done in the same place, preferably in a quiet room where you can spend about 5 to 10 minutes uninterrupted. You can be as general or specific as you consider necessary. With greater self-awareness, self-talk becomes more appropriate. Self-talk can be either positive or negative. Knowing your position on the EPS allows you to determine whether important decisions should be made. One tends to make more intelligent and better decisions when their emotions are within or closer to the happiness Zone on the EPS.

Gratitude Journaling

Among the various types of journaling, gratitude journaling is particularly useful.

Gratitude journaling allows one to combat negativity and stress and restore the positive mindset you need. This occurs by allowing individuals to positively reframe stressful life events and to try to determine their meaning.

In giving gratitude, one cannot help showing appreciation for the entity for which they give thanks. In a subtle manner, since they are giving thanks for the receipt of an item, they are surreptitiously showing approval for the receipt of their gift. It is difficult to show appreciation and approval for an item that you do not admire, so by showing gratitude you hint at your admiration of the item. There is inevitably a level of attention you give to any item for which you say thanks. Attention is thus given to the item for which you give thanks. Organically, gratitude causes synchronized activation in several brain areas. Gratitude boosts the neurotransmitter serotonin and activates the brain stem to produce dopamine. Dopamine is our brain's pleasure chemical. Hence by saying thanks, it evokes some pleasure or pleasant feelings. Keeping a gratitude Journal causes less stress, improves the quality of sleep, and builds emotional awareness. It also improves your relationships and facilitates your ability to create new relationships. You are less irritable and aggressive. Improvement occurs in both your confidence and self-esteem with gratitude journaling.

Thoughts and Their Triggers

With a heightened sense of self awareness, you are now able to determine your location on the EPS. You also become aware of your self-talk and their nature. Self-talk is broadly placed in two categories. (a) positive self-talk and negative self-talk. "Positive self-talk says Jantz, 2019, is showing yourself some self-compassion and understanding who you are and what you have been through. With positive self-talk our internal narrative switches to ideas like, I can do better, or I choose to learn from my mistakes and not be held back by them. Positive self-talk is the encouraging, uplifting, and supportive way you talk to yourself, much like showing self-compassion. Positive self-talk is therefore motivating and can give you the drive to help you acquire your dreams.

We have recognized the importance of Focus in impacting our emotional health and our position on the EPS. Focus plays an integral role in acquiring gifts from the universe which you request. It also plays a vital role in determining our position on our EPS. Every effort should be made to seek out practices which can intensify our focus. The value of Journaling cannot be ignored in this regard.

Negative Self-Talk

It is more common in certain states, for example, if you are depressed or low on confidence, you are already dealing with many negative feelings and thoughts, in keeping with the law of attraction, negative self-talk becomes easy, and are composed of most of your thoughts.

According to mayo clinic staff 2022; there are about eight kinds of negative thinking patterns of which we need to be aware so that we can identify them and evict them from our thought processes because negative self-talk is self-damaging. These are (a) filtering, (b) personalizing, (c)blaming, (d) catastrophizing, (e) magnifying, (f) should 'statements',(g) perfectionism, (h) polarizing. Looking at these processes, you may wonder whether they apply to you, so to clarify, I will give a brief description of each process.

In filtering, a person focusses on the negatives associated with a condition, and completely ignores the positives. For example, after completing a day's work, in which much was achieved but there is still a lot to be done, you instead of focusing on the accomplished task, you 'beat' yourself up lamenting that you can never get all that is required done.

Personalizing on the other hand means that you blame yourself for any mishaps even if you are not at fault.

Blaming on the other hand is the exact opposite of personalizing, one with that predisposition tends to blame others while you completely exonerate yourself from culpability.

In catastrophizing, one assumes and expects the worst of any situation.

Perfectionism though is unrealistic in its foundation, so people who are perfectionists tend to set lofty standards which are unattainable.

When they fail to attain these standards, they get angry and view themselves as failures.

In magnifying people tend to make situations bigger than they are, akin to making mountains out of a molehill.

The should statements are thoughts about what you should or should not be doing. These statements can be unrealistic and induce a significant amount of guilt in these people.

In polarizing, people tend to see things as either black or white, not grey areas; something is either good or bad. It may mean you saying to yourself that you are not good enough, if you fail at a task.

Planful Time Management

With planful time management your focus is better, there is more structure to your activities. The processes are organized and so the chance for success is improved. This approach is encouraged to facilitate your successes and to reduce failure. Simultaneously, it reduces stress and in combination with a healthy dose of positive self-talk; it will positively impact your spirit leading to your rise up your EPS.

Life is complex with a continuous stream of challenges that we must face. We always have a choice in how we emerge in the face of these challenges. We hope that we are providing you with useful tools which you may adopt to ensure you live your best life and grow into your excellence.

Reflection:

What is your position on your EPS?

How do your thoughts influence how you feel about yourself?

When you are not having a good day, what thoughts come easiest to you?

Have you been able to identify occasions when your self-talk is negative?

How have you addressed your negative self-talk

How do you make the transition from negative self-talk to positive self-talk?

How does that make you feel?

_____

_____

_____

_____

_____

_____

_____

_____

_____

_____

Chapter 21: Bringing It All Together

"Everyone has inside of him a piece of good news. The good news is that you don't know how great you can be! How much you can love! What you can accomplish! And what your potential is!" – Anne Frank

The Complexity

It is evident that you are much more complex than meets the eye. You are more than just your physical body. You are a multilayered and interesting entity. It is up to you to develop the triune, '**you'**, in whatever capacity you wish. I must remind you that whichever point of the journey you are on in your life, it is not too late to start from where you are. Willing or not, change is the only constant taking place within you and around you, thus, you have a choice. You can be an active participant and marshal those changes to serve in your revival. Or you can be a passive attendant and simply observe the changes as they happen year after year. The choice is YOURS and yours alone. Do you wish to be a bystander in your life, or an active participant?...

A bystander gives up their ability to choose, either willingly or it is taken from him. Either way, the bystander lacks the control of their destiny, has sacrificed their authority and ability to guide their life to a desired location. When you choose to be a bystander in your life, you become complacent and just accept all that happens to your body, mind, and spirit with each passing year.

An active participant, on the other hand, retains a vested interest in the direction of their journey, creates goals and targets their approach to the desired destiny. They remain aware of how they are growing and developing in their body, mind, and spirit, and they remain committed to growing each part of themself. To simply exist is not their idea of how they want to live their life.

After thoroughly examining the triune of which you are composed, I trust you feel empowered to play a more active role in your revival and you now have the required tools for growing into your excellence. You now have the tools to nourish, adapt to appropriate environments and protect each component of yourself from the negative ever-present aspects of life that can adversely affect your person. It is now up to you to commit to your revival and add years to your life and life to your years while you grow into your excellence.

Any positive activity you perform has an impact on all components of yourself. A great example of this is the act of physical exercise. When you exercise you are strengthening the muscular and cardiovascular systems and contributing to your weight management. Additionally, when we move our body, our brain also releases endorphins which improve our mood and give us an emotional "high", affecting both the mind and the spirit. It results in the appropriate movement along our Emotional Positioning system. Every action has a reaction, no matter which component of yourself is working. They are all intertwined, and every action counts.

No one tries to run away from things that are good for them. Rather they run full steam ahead into them and embrace the great possibility of living a full and rich life! This is what I wish for you and why

I wanted to share this revival process. We are triunes, and we must have all three components of ourselves working in harmony to really reap the rewards of your efforts.

Reflection:

What is the biggest take-away I have personally learned about my body?

My mind?

My Spirit?

What was the biggest "ah-ha!" moment in reading this book?

What is something I can start working on right away to serve me positively on my growth into my excellence?

What is the one thing I would want to share with someone I love?

_____

_____

_____

_____

_____

_____

_____

_____

Final Thoughts...

There is a potency which results when all three elements are appropriately aligned which forces the universe to take note and create a healthier and more dynamic life for you. My favorite example of this is my paternal Grandmother. She lived to the grand old age of 115 years! (She was even recognized as the eldest woman on earth for years.) What was her secret you may ask? It wasn't simple luck, or great genetic make-up. She was active and vibrant with unwavering faith. You could see that all parts of her fed each other to create a synergy and vibrancy to her life. In my mind her life bore testimony to the BMS ecosystem thus adding years to her life and life to her years.

Further evidence emerges from the nun's study that gives a broad insight into tools which convey longer and productive lives. In this study, 1,932 Nuns were asked to write biochemical sketches of their lives. Based on their sketches, the Nuns were placed into four groups. Nuns whose sketch revealed the most positive and optimistic feeling were placed in group A. In group D were those whose sketches revealed the least optimism and were the most negative, the other two groups were in between these two extremes. After 85 years, 95% of the Nuns in group A were still living active lives whereas only 34% of the nuns in group D were alive; after 90 years, 54% of the Nuns in Group A were still alive and only 11% of those in group D were alive. That is remarkable, isn't it? Is this the result of luck or good genes? Surely it could be neither because the only thing the nuns in group A had which the nuns in group D did not have is a difference in optimism and positivity. It was their spirit and mindset that truly set them apart, and as we have discussed I am sure that because our three components of body, mind and spirit are interconnected, the positivity of their emotions and the optimism of their mind most certainly affected the whole of their lives. The potent forces of the Universe will take note of your efforts and reward you with years to your life and life to your years while facilitating your growth into your excellence.

The value of this phenomenon is currently explored in the positive psychology movement. This movement has thus far revealed the countless benefits to be had on your longevity, health, and happiness through positive thinking.

My deepest passion and one of my life missions is to share this process of revival with as many people as I can! You *deserve* to live your best life well into your golden years. Imagine being able to see your grandchildren grow into independent adults and to spend quality time with your great grandchildren?... It is possible!

I look forward to connecting more with you in the future. Take good care of your body, mind, and spirit, and in turn, enjoy the benefits of living the most vibrant days of your life yet!

Dr. Harris Phillip is available as a guest speaker, for interviews and for seminars, consultations, and workshops. Look forward to his future series of seminars and his workshops, "Don't Just Tell Me, SHOW ME." To find out more and to book please check out his website:

www.philburnacademy.com

Do not hesitate to pop him an email if you have any questions or are interested in engaging his services!

Acknowledgements

Certainly, Rome was not built in a day, and so I pause to appreciate all who have in myriad ways helped me to become who I am today. I am acutely aware and believe that all that I am and ever hope to become was not simply born out of some innate characteristic but instead is a product of a multiplicity of influences whom I acknowledge and to whom I say thanks.

On reflection, I genuinely acknowledge and say thanks to everyone who has contributed to my existence to date. Every encounter, every interaction, every challenge, every resistance was but an additional building block in my personal development.

To my informal teachers, my earliest educators, my immediate family, parents and siblings, your efforts at teaching me early the differences between right and wrong and protecting me from myself is a major reason why I am here today and so for that I thank you.

From my teachers at all levels of my formal education beginning from my earliest kindergarten days through to elementary school, through to high school, college, and university, you all made a significant contribution to my growth and training and to you I extend my gratitude.

To my various students at high school and university levels in the Caribbean, USA, and the UK. Thanks for your contribution to my education and growth. Each of you in your own distinct and individual way made a definite impact on me and who I have become today. Because of your contributions, I continue to grow year after year not only as a teacher but as a human being.

To my patients, your confidence and trust in me, coupled with the opportunity you gave me to be involved in your care, has served me well and for your unique contributions to my growth, I extend my gratitude.

To my acquaintances and friends, I say thanks for your friendships and interactions over the years. Through various discussions and conversations, you have made an indelible impact on me and continue to leave an imprint on my person.

To my current life coaches and mentors, I am eternally grateful for your continued invaluable contributions. I will continue to strive to ensure that your guidance and training have not been in vain.

As you can see, I have stayed clear from name calling. I have always found that to be divisive and essentially double edged. My aim is to level the platform of individual contribution since everyone with whom I traversed paths has contributed to my growth in some way. I see myself as being carried around on the shoulders of all those with whom I come into contact, and I acknowledge everyone no matter how small or large your impact.

My deepest and heartfelt thanks… everyone.

Biography – Long

Harris E. Phillip, MD has been practicing medicine for three plus decades, with a focus as a consultant Obstetrician and Gynecologist. Harris received a BSc (summa cum laude honors) in Chemistry and a MSc in chemistry, before proceeding to spend a year in the PHD program in Biochemistry/Organic Chemistry at Texas A&M University. He also possesses an MBBS degree, Doctor of Medicine (DM) degree and a master's degree in law (LLM degree). Harris is a fellow of both the American College of Obstetricians and Gynecologists (USA) and the Royal college of Obstetricians and Gynecologists (UK), and he is a former Chairman and Vice-chairman of the junior fellows of the American College of Obstetricians and Gynecologists.

Harris' work is widely published in international medical journals, and he has contributed to an array of print and online educational tools in the medical field. He is currently a reviewer for 11 international journals and helps to determine what is medically acceptable and publishable in those journals. Beyond his own practice, he has also lectured nursing students, nurses, midwifery students, midwives, medical students, as well as junior and senior medical doctors for more than 20 years.

His current passion lies in helping you live your best life through understanding that when your body, mind and spirit are in harmony, you will truly be able to lead your best life and grow into your excellence!

www.philburnacademy.com

Biography – Short

With more than 30 years as a practicing MD and over 20 years lecturing health care professionals, Dr. Harris Phillip is passionate about you achieving your highest level of health which will ensure that you live your best life. He believes that not only do you have to take care of your body, but also your mind and spirit to achieve a total state of wellbeing that will add years to your life and life to your years!

www.philburnacademy.com

www.ingramcontent.com/pod-product-compliance
Lightning Source LLC
Chambersburg PA
CBHW062126020426
42335CB00013B/1111

* 9 7 8 1 9 6 2 9 4 8 4 9 4 *